Childhood Obesity

T0314450

About the Authors

Denise E. Wilfley, PhD, is the Scott Rudolph University Professor of Psychiatry, Medicine, Pediatrics, and Psychological & Brain Sciences, and Director of the Weight Management and Eating Disorders Program at Washington University School of Medicine. She has dedicated her career to researching the etiology, prevention, and treatment of obesity and eating disorders in children and adults, and to the dissemination and implementation of evidence-based practices into clinical settings.

John R. Best, PhD, is a research associate within the Faculty of Medicine at the University of British Columbia in Vancouver, Canada. With a background in developmental psychology, he studies lifestyle behaviors that promote cognitive and brain health across the lifespan, as well as the cognitive, neural, and environmental factors that contribute to healthy choice behavior.

Jodi Cahill Holland, PhD, RD, is a registered dietitian. After completing a postdoctoral fellowship at Washington University in St. Louis' School of Medicine conducting research in the field of childhood obesity, she relocated to Texas where she is happily applying her knowledge to the raising of her two young children.

Dorothy J. Van Buren, PhD, retired in 2018 from the position of Associate Professor within the Department of Psychiatry at Washington University in St. Louis School of Medicine. She passed away shortly before publication of this book. For the past 27 years, she had served as a clinical psychologist, supervisor, and researcher in the field of childhood obesity and disordered eating. She is remembered by many for her leadership, compassion, patience, kindness and intelligence. She is dearly missed by her family as well as students, staff, faculty and colleagues. She is survived by her husband, Martin, and her two daughters, Medora and Miranda.

Advances in Psychotherapy – Evidence-Based Practice

Series Editor
Danny Wedding, PhD, MPH, Saybrook University, Oakland, CA

Associate Editors
Larry Beutler, PhD, Professor, Palo Alto University / Pacific Graduate School of Psychology, Palo Alto, CA
Kenneth E. Freedland, PhD, Professor of Psychiatry and Psychology, Washington University School of Medicine, St. Louis, MO
Linda C. Sobell, PhD, ABPP, Professor, Center for Psychological Studies, Nova Southeastern University, Ft. Lauderdale, FL
David A. Wolfe, PhD, Adjunct Professor, Faculty of Education, Western University, London, ON

The basic objective of this series is to provide therapists with practical, evidence-based treatment guidance for the most common disorders seen in clinical practice – and to do so in a reader-friendly manner. Each book in the series is both a compact "how-to" reference on a particular disorder for use by professional clinicians in their daily work and an ideal educational resource for students as well as for practice-oriented continuing education.

The most important feature of the books is that they are practical and easy to use: All are structured similarly and all provide a compact and easy-to-follow guide to all aspects that are relevant in real-life practice. Tables, boxed clinical "pearls," marginal notes, and summary boxes assist orientation, while checklists provide tools for use in daily practice.

Continuing Education Credits

Psychologists and other healthcare providers may earn five continuing education credits for reading the books in the *Advances in Psychotherapy* series and taking a multiple-choice exam. This continuing education program is a partnership of Hogrefe Publishing and the National Register of Health Service Psychologists. Details are available at https://us.hogrefe.com/cenatreg

The National Register of Health Service Psychologists is approved by the American Psychological Association to sponsor continuing education for psychologists. The National Register maintains responsibility for this program and its content.

Childhood Obesity

Denise E. Wilfley
Center for Healthy Weight and Wellness and
Department of Psychiatry, Washington University
School of Medicine, St. Louis, MO

John R. Best
Djavad Mowafaghian Centre for Brain Health,
University of British Columbia, Vancouver, BC, Canada

Jodi Cahill Holland
Austin, TX

Dorothy J. Van Buren
Center for Healthy Weight and Wellness,
Washington University School of Medicine, St. Louis, MO

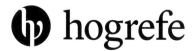

Library of Congress Cataloging in Publication information for the print version of this book is available via the Library of Congress Marc Database under the Library of Congress Control Number 2018935330

Library and Archives Canada Cataloguing in Publication

Wilfley, Denise E., 1960-, author
    Childhood obesity / Denise E. Wilfley, Department of Psychiatry, Washington University School of Medicine, St. Louis, MO, John R. Best, Djavad Mowafaghian Centre for Brain Health, University of British Columbia, Vancouver, BC, Canada, Jodi Cahill Holland, Austin, TX, Dorothy J. Van Buren, Weight Management and Eating Disorders Research Lab, Washington University School of Medicine, St. Louis, MO.

(Advances in psychotherapy--evidence-based practice ; v. 39)
Includes bibliographical references.
Issued in print and electronic formats.
ISBN 978-0-88937-406-5 (softcover).--ISBN 978-1-61676-406-7 (PDF).--
ISBN 978-1-61334-406-4 (EPUB)

    1. Obesity in children. 2. Obesity--Treatment. 3. Overweight children--Family relationships.
I. Title. II. Series: Advances in psychotherapy--evidence-based practice ; v. 39

RJ399.C6W53 2018   618.92'398   C2018-901255-2
                                              C2018-901256-0

The authors and publisher have made every effort to ensure that the information contained in this text is in accord with the current state of scientific knowledge, recommendations, and practice at the time of publication. In spite of this diligence, errors cannot be completely excluded. Also, due to changing regulations and continuing research, information may become outdated at any point. The authors and publisher disclaim any responsibility for any consequences which may follow from the use of information presented in this book.

Registered trademarks are not noted specifically as such in this publication. The use of descriptive names, registered names, and trademarks does not imply, even in the absence of a specific statement, that such names are exempt from the relevant protective laws and regulations and therefore free for general use.

Cover image: © kali9 – iStock.com

The cover image is an agency photo depicting models. Use of the photo on this publication does not imply any connection between the content of this publication and any person depicted in the cover image.

© 2019 by Hogrefe Publishing
http://www.hogrefe.com

PUBLISHING OFFICES

USA: Hogrefe Publishing Corporation, 7 Bulfinch Place, Suite 202, Boston, MA 02114
              Phone (866) 823-4726, Fax (617) 354-6875; E-mail customerservice@hogrefe.com
EUROPE: Hogrefe Publishing GmbH, Merkelstr. 3, 37085 Göttingen, Germany
              Phone +49 551 99950-0, Fax +49 551 99950-111; E-mail publishing@hogrefe.com

SALES & DISTRIBUTION

USA: Hogrefe Publishing, Customer Services Department,
              30 Amberwood Parkway, Ashland, OH 44805
              Phone (800) 228-3749, Fax (419) 281-6883; E-mail customerservice@hogrefe.com
UK: Hogrefe Publishing, c/o Marston Book Services Ltd., 160 Eastern Ave.,
              Milton Park, Abingdon, OX14 4SB, UK
              Phone +44 1235 465577, Fax +44 1235 465556; E-mail direct.orders@marston.co.uk
EUROPE: Hogrefe Publishing, Merkelstr. 3, 37085 Göttingen, Germany
              Phone +49 551 99950-0, Fax +49 551 99950-111; E-mail publishing@hogrefe.com

OTHER OFFICES

CANADA: Hogrefe Publishing, 660 Eglinton Ave. East, Suite 119-514, Toronto, Ontario, M4G 2K2
SWITZERLAND: Hogrefe Publishing, Länggass-Strasse 76, 3012 Bern

Hogrefe Publishing
Incorporated and registered in the Commonwealth of Massachusetts, USA, and in Göttingen, Lower Saxony, Germany

No part of this book may be reproduced, stored in a retrieval system or transmitted, in any form or by any means, electronic, mechanical, photocopying, microfilming, recording or otherwise, without written permission from the publisher.

Printed and bound in the USA

ISBN 978-0-88937-406-5 (print) • ISBN 978-1-61676-406-7 (PDF) • ISBN 978-1-61334-406-4 (EPUB)
http://doi.org/10.1027/00406-000

Preface

This compact desk reference is ideal for busy clinicians who treat pediatric patients with obesity, providing a comprehensive summary of the current state of knowledge and evidence-based recommendations on this important public health concern. Childhood obesity affects one in every six children and as much as one in every five ethnic minority children. Despite its being a widespread affliction, misunderstandings of the origins and resolution of obesity abound. Weight loss gimmicks and health claims oversimplify weight gain and appeal to desperate families by offering pseudoscience and quick fixes that don't work. In reality, obesity develops from a number of complex and varied environmental, genetic, and psychological factors, which present differently between individuals. Successful treatment of the pediatric patient is also complex, requiring time-intensive, evidence-based care delivered by a multidisciplinary team. In the following chapters, the reader will find the most current scientific understanding of obesity and be equipped to help guide patients to appropriate and effective treatment modalities.

The book is divided into five chapters. The first chapter defines obesity and describes the prevalence both globally and in the US. A report of the consequences of untreated obesity as it tracks into adulthood, and the associated physical and psychosocial comorbidities, is provided. In this chapter, the reader will also find the current definitions and methods used to screen for childhood obesity. Chapter 2 explores the theoretical models of the causes of obesity, including behavioral causes such as eating behaviors and physical inactivity; appetitive traits such as impulsivity, motivation to consume palatable food, and satiety responsiveness; environmental causes such as the family and built environments; and genetic influences. A discussion of behavioral economics and its relevance to the adoption of treatment strategies is also included. In Chapter 3, diagnostic criteria and individual and familial factors that are predictive of weight loss treatment are provided. Chapter 4 describes current treatment guidelines and approaches to treatment including family-based treatment, social facilitation maintenance, pharmacotherapy, and surgical procedures. In particular, a family-based treatment method is outlined which is best supported by the evidence and which meets the recommendations of the American Academy of Pediatrics, US Preventive Services Task Force, and other organizations. Clinicians can use the copyable resources provided in the Appendix to initiate this recommended treatment strategy: a sample session outline; self-monitoring forms to track eating, sleeping, and activity behaviors; and a tool to evaluate socioenvironmental contexts to facilitate individualized treatment planning. The reader will also find a discussion of prevention strategies, current understanding of the mechanisms of action for successful outcomes, and the efficacy of and prognosis for multicomponent behavioral interventions. Problems that may arise in treatment implementation and multicultural issues are also described. Chapter 5 provides a detailed case vignette of a 12-year-old girl and her mother.

The book can be read cover-to-cover or as a reference manual to fulfill an immediate need to identify specific information. Because of the complex nature of obesity, treatment is fraught with challenges. These challenges require a persistent and focused team effort. Patients require education, social support, behavioral and family therapy, and in some cases medical supervision. The multicomponent treatment protocol is intensive, but the health and psychosocial benefits can last a lifetime.

Dedication

Dedicated to the children, families, and interventionists who participated in obesity research trials. Without you there would be no evidence upon which to base our treatments.

Acknowledgments

Denise Wilfley would like to thank the National Institutes of Health, whose support made it possible to study the treatment of childhood obesity and to provide treatment for so many wonderful children and families. In addition, she would like to thank Dr. Leonard Epstein, a pioneering colleague in the field of childhood obesity, with whom she has collaborated for over 25 years on childhood obesity treatment studies. She would also like to acknowledge the wisdom she has acquired from her family, especially her mother, Arlene Wilfley, and her late father, Donald Gene Wilfley. She also wishes to express deep gratitude to her husband, Rob Welch, and children, Wil, Emma, and Ella, for their unending support and inspiration.

John R. Best and Jodi Cahill Holland would like to thank their professional mentors for their guidance and support.

Dorothy Van Buren, who sadly passed away shortly before the publication of this book, expressed her gratitude for the loving support of her husband, Martin West, and daughters, Medora and Miranda, during the writing of this book.

The authors wish to acknowledge the research and clinical teams, including Mackenzie Brown, for invaluable help in compiling this book and for providing insightful observations over the years.

Contents

1

Description

1.1   Terminology

Obesity is not currently included in the *Diagnostic and Statistical Manual of Mental Disorders,* 5th edition (DSM-5; American Psychiatric Association, 2013). Deliberations for inclusion were allowed because of the body of evidence documenting associations and similar behaviors and brain patterns, between obesity and many other psychiatric disorders. However, the Eating Disorders Work Group of the task force concluded that there is insufficient evidence to include obesity in the DSM-5, because of the heterogeneity observed across the condition and the incompletely understood etiology (Marcus & Wildes, 2012). In contrast, obesity is formally recognized as a disease by the American Medical Association (Pollack, 2013) and the Obesity Society (Allison et al., 2008).

1.2   Definition

The World Health Organization (WHO) defines *overweight* and *obesity* as "abnormal or excessive fat accumulation that may impair health" (World Health Organization, 2014). Identification of children with excess weight is a challenge due to the influences of child age, sex, pubertal status, and race/ethnicity on body composition. To account for these factors and the growth rate in children, the US Centers for Disease Control and Prevention (CDC) and the WHO have developed age- and sex-specific growth charts, which were updated in 2000 and 2006, respectively (Borghi et al., 2006; Kuczmarski et al., 2002). Definitions for obesity in childhood have been issued by the WHO (de Onis et al., 2007), CDC (Kuczmarski et al., 2002), and International Task Force on Obesity (IOTF) (Cole, Bellizzi, Flegal, & Dietz, 2000) (Table 1).

Child BMI is used to identify overweight and obesity in children

Child weight status is determined first by calculating *body mass index* (BMI), defined as a child's weight in kilograms divided by the child's height in meters squared, and second, by comparing the child's current BMI with the age- and sex-specific reference values. IOTF cutoffs are based on combined international reference data from Brazil, Great Britain, Hong Kong, The Netherlands, Singapore, and the US (Cole et al., 2000) and are not intended for clinical use. More information regarding the use of BMI in the identification of child overweight and obesity is provided in Section 1.7.

Table 1
Definitions of Childhood and Adult Overweight and Obesity

Source	Age	Overweight	Obese	Underweight
CDC	2–19	BMI ≥ 85th percentile and < 95th percentile	BMI ≥ 95th percentile	BMI < 5th percentile
WHO	0–5	BMI > 2 standard deviations above the WHO growth standard median	BMI > 3 standard deviations above the WHO growth standard median	BMI < 2 standard deviations below the WHO growth standard median
WHO	5–9	BMI > 1 standard deviation above the WHO growth standard median	BMI > 2 standard deviations above the WHO growth standard median	BMI < 2 standard deviations below the WHO growth standard median
International Obesity Task Force[a]	2–18	International age- and sex-specific BMI cutoff points that correspond to the adult definition of ≥ 25 BMI	International age- and sex-specific BMI cutoff points that correspond to the adult definition of ≥ 30 BMI	International age- and sex-specific BMI cutoff points that correspond to the < 18.5 or < 17 BMI adult criteria are suggested, but these points need validation
CDC, WHO	Adults	25.0 ≤ BMI ≤ 29.9	BMI ≥ 30.0 **Subcategories** Grade 1: BMI 30–35 Grade 2: BMI 35–40 Grade 3: BMI ≥ 40	BMI < 18.5

Note. Body mass index (BMI) is defined as weight in kilograms divided by height in meters squared. CDC = US Centers for Disease Control and Prevention; WHO = World Health Organization.
[a]Not intended for clinical use.

1.3   Epidemiology

The global prevalence of obesity has risen dramatically in recent decades (Swinburn et al., 2011). Although it is difficult to directly compare obesity prevalence among youths of different countries, due to differing definitions of obesity, childhood obesity tends to be more prevalent in the US than in other developed countries (Ogden, Carroll, Kit, & Flegal, 2012). In the US, the national rate of childhood obesity is 18.5% for children ages 2–19 (The State of Obesity, 2017), indicating that the rate of childhood obesity has tripled over the past 40 years. Other developed countries (Swinburn et al., 2011) and even developing countries in South America, Africa, and Southeast Asia (Gupta, Goel, Shah, & Misra, 2012) have also shown increases in childhood obesity prevalence. Increases in childhood obesity are especially pronounced in the Gulf Arab states, such as the United Arab Emirates (Malik & Bakir, 2007). Globally among preschool children (< 5 years old), 43 million to 35 million in developing countries alone were estimated to have overweight or obesity in 2010 (de Onis, Blossner, & Borghi, 2010).

Both in the US and globally, sex and age differences in childhood obesity have been observed, but such differences are not always consistent. The most recent report from the US National Health and Nutrition Examination Survey (NHANES) suggested there were increases in obesity prevalence among male youths (aged 2–19 years) but not female youths, during the first decade of the 21st century (Ogden et al., 2012). However, sex differences are inconsistent when examined globally. In some countries, rates are higher among female youths (e.g., India, Saudi Arabia, and South Africa), whereas in others, rates are higher among male youths (e.g., Beirut, Sri Lanka, and Malaysia; Gupta et

Nearly 1 in 5 US children and adolescents have obesity

Childhood obesity rates have increased in many developed and developing countries

Table 2
Prevalence of Childhood Obesity (BMI ≥ 95th Percentile) by Age, Sex, and Race/Ethnicity in the US

Race/Ethnicity	Age group		
	2–5 years	6–11 years	12–19 years
Males			
Hispanic	17.8%	23.9%	26.5%
Non-Hispanic Black	20.5%	29.5%	22.6%
Non-Hispanic White	11.9%	16.8%	17.5%
Females			
Hispanic	14.6%	21.0%	19.8%
Non-Hispanic Black	17.0%	27.8%	24.8%
Non-Hispanic White	6.0%	10.7%	14.7%

Note. Based on Ogden et al., 2012

al., 2012). In terms of age, obesity prevalence is typically higher among older children and adolescents as compared with preschool-aged children, and differences among older children and adolescents are often small or negligible. This is a trend seen in the US and internationally (Gupta et al., 2012; Ogden et al., 2012).

In the US, there are persistent differences in childhood obesity based on race and ethnicity. Obesity is more prevalent among Hispanic children and adolescents and non-Hispanic Black children and adolescents, in comparison with non-Hispanic White children and adolescents (Ogden et al., 2012). Table 2 provides a breakdown of childhood obesity rates in the US based on age, sex, and race/ethnicity.

1.4   Course and Prognosis

1.4.1   Obesity Tracking Into Adulthood

Children with obesity are at heightened risk of becoming adults with obesity

Left untreated, childhood obesity tracks into adulthood, and the risk of tracking increases with age and obesity severity. In a large study of multiple longitudinal cohorts from several developed countries, researchers found that among children (aged 3–19 years) who were affected by overweight or obesity ($\geq$ 85th BMI percentile), nearly 65% developed or remained affected by obesity as adults (age range 23–46 years), whereas among those children with obesity ($\geq$ 95th BMI percentile), over 82% remained affected by obesity as adults (Juonala et al., 2011). Others have concluded that children younger than 12 years with overweight or obesity are at least twice as likely to develop overweight or obesity as adults, and that adolescents with overweight and obesity are at even greater risk of becoming adults with overweight or obesity (Singh, Mulder, Twisk, van Mechelen, & Chinapaw, 2008). Overall, there is strong evidence that children with overweight and obesity are at heightened risk of obesity in adulthood compared with their leaner counterparts, and that this risk increases with childhood obesity severity and age. These findings may reflect the persistence of obesogenic habits (e.g., excess calorie consumption and sedentary behavior) into adulthood, and that these unhealthy habits become more ingrained with age.

1.4.2   Future Medical Problems

Childhood obesity is associated with many future negative health consequences

Children with overweight and obesity are at greater risk of experiencing increased medical problems as adults (Park, Falconer, Viner, & Kinra, 2012). These negative health consequences appear to be most closely related to cardiometabolic functioning but may also include increased risk of several types of cancer. Children with obesity are at especially high risk of developing metabolic syndrome as adults, which refers to the presence of a constellation of metabolic risk factors that predispose individuals to future coronary heart disease, diabetes, and stroke. A brief description of individual risk factors that are part of metabolic syndrome can be found in Table 3. Generally, metabolic syndrome is believed to be present when an individual presents with at least three of these risk factors.

The increased risk for metabolic syndrome and cardiovascular disease as adults may be explained in part by the tracking of obesity into adulthood – that is, children with obesity might be at greater risk for disease as adults because they are also more likely to have obesity as adults. This is perhaps most clearly shown by the aforementioned study by Juonala and colleagues (2011). These researchers compared four groups of individuals: Group 1 included those individuals who were within a healthy weight range both as children and as adults, Group 2 included those individuals who had obesity as children but not when assessed as adults, Group 3 included those who had obesity both as children and as adults, and Group 4 included those who did not have obesity as children but did have obesity as adults. In comparison with those who were persistently at a healthy weight from childhood to mid-adulthood (Group 1), both those who persistently evidenced obesity from childhood to adulthood (Group 3) and those who did not have obesity as children but did as adults (Group 4) were at heightened risk of having metabolic syndrome as adults (i.e., approximately 1.7 times more likely to have at least one component of metabolic syndrome), whereas those who had obesity only as children (Group 2) had no greater risk than the group with persistently healthy weights (Group 1). This suggests that children with obesity who normalize their weight by mid-adulthood may diminish or even eliminate their risk for metabolic syndrome as adults. This is an encouraging message for clinicians because it suggests that children with overweight and obesity are not fated to have cardiometabolic disease later in life. Given proper treatment to help them normalize their

Children with obesity who become normal weight adults reduce their risk of medical complications

Table 3
Risk Factors for Metabolic Syndrome

Risk factor	Description
High fasting blood glucose	High blood sugar may be an early sign of diabetes development.
Hypertension	Hypertension refers to high blood pressure and indicates that the force of blood on the arterial walls is elevated. Hypertension can damage the heart and lead to plaque buildup.
High triglycerides	Triglycerides are a type of fat found in the blood that can raise your risk of heart disease.
Low HDL cholesterol	High-density lipoprotein (HDL) is often called the "good" cholesterol because it aids in the removal of other cholesterols from arteries. Low HDL cholesterol increases the risk for heart disease.
Large waist circumference	A large waistline is indicative of excess abdominal fat, which is a much stronger risk factor for heart disease and diabetes than fat found in other parts of the body.

Note. Based on http://www.nhlbi.nih.gov/health/health-topics/metabolic-syndrome

weight, children with overweight and obesity can be as healthy in later life as their peers with healthy weight.

1.4.3   Premature Mortality

An analysis of multiple studies demonstrated that adult obesity, especially Grades 2 and 3 (BMI between 35 and 40, and BMI ≥ 40, respectively), is associated with significantly higher all-cause mortality relative to normal weight (Flegal, Kit, Orpana, & Graubard, 2013). Specifically, adults with Grades 2 or 3 obesity had 1.3 times the risk of all-cause premature mortality compared with their counterparts with healthy weight. A systematic review looking across the lifespan found that childhood obesity was associated with an increased rate of all-cause mortality, with several of the larger studies showing an increased risk of between 40% and 60%; however, the authors of this review note that this effect may be attenuated by taking into account obesity in adulthood (Park et al., 2012). Stated another way, childhood obesity may be linked to premature mortality because children with obesity are more likely to become adults with obesity, and it is really the obesity in adulthood that contributes to premature mortality. In line with the results in the study by Juonala et al. (2011), these findings suggest that normalization of weight in childhood can significantly diminish the premature mortality risk associated with obesity.

1.5   Differential Diagnosis

The majority of presenting cases of obesity in childhood can be attributed to lifestyle factors (diet and physical activity). However, in rare instances, secondary obesity can occur as a result of a variety of conditions and treatments. A list of conditions that may also present with obesity can be found in Table 4.

1.6   Comorbidities

1.6.1   Physical Comorbidities

Childhood obesity can have immediate negative effects on physical and psychosocial health

Childhood obesity not only has long-term health consequences, but is also associated with several immediate and wide-reaching complications (Ludwig, 2007). Many of the cardiometabolic effects mentioned above are not necessarily delayed until adulthood, and symptoms such as high blood pressure, high blood sugar, and insulin resistance can develop as early as childhood, especially in cases of severe obesity. Other short-term effects include increased blood pressure inside the skull (pseudotumor cerebri), which can result in vision loss; breathing disorders (e.g., sleep apnea and asthma); and discoloration of the skin around folds and creases (acanthosis nigricans). All of these physical effects can negatively affect the quality of the child's life, as they may contribute to restricted activity as well as promote teasing and ostracism by peers.

Table 4
Conditions and Treatments Associated With Secondary Obesity

Risk factor	Description
Endocrine	Cushing's syndrome Hypothyroidism Growth hormone deficiency Hyperinsulinemia Pseudohypoparathyroidism (Albright's hereditary dystrophy)
Central nervous system disorders or brain damage	Hypothalamic tumor Surgery Trauma Postinflammation Postchemotherapy
Genetic syndromes	Prader-Labhart-Willi syndrome Alström syndrome Bardet-Biedl syndrome Carpenter syndrome Cohen syndrome Smith-Magenis syndrome Fragile X syndrome SIM1 mutation WAGR syndrome
Pharmacological agents	Insulin therapy (or insulin secretagogues) Glucocorticoids Hormonal contraceptives Psychotropic medications (clozapine, olanzapine, risperidone) Mood stabilizers (lithium) Tricyclic antidepressants (amitriptyline, imipramine, nortriptyline) Anticonvulsants (valproic acid, gabapentin, carbamazepine) Antihypertensives (propranolol, clonidine) Antihistamines
Large waist circumference	A large waistline is indicative of excess abdominal fat, which is a much stronger risk factor for heart disease and diabetes than fat found in other parts of the body.

1.6.2   Psychosocial Comorbidities

In addition to these negative physiological effects to the organ systems, there are a number of negative psychosocial comorbidities associated with childhood obesity that range from internalizing (e.g., depression) to externalizing (e.g., impulsive behavior) emotional and behavioral disorders and include deficits in social functioning and academic achievement (Gable, Krull, & Chang, 2012; Puder & Munsch, 2010). Table 5 provides an overview of these comorbidities.

Table 5
Examples of Psychosocial Comorbidities of Childhood Obesity and
Their Assessment

General domain	Psychosocial comorbidity and definition	Assessment instruments or methods
Internalizing or externalizing disorders	**Anxiety disorders** – persistent anxiety that interferes with normal functioning; extreme avoidance. **Depression** – depressed mood, loss of interest or pleasure in activities, decreased energy. **Impulsive behavior** – acting without thinking ahead, preference for immediate rewards irrespective of long-term consequences. **Attention-deficit/ hyperactivity disorder (ADHD)** – stable pattern ($\geq$ 6 months) of inattentive or hyperactive/ impulsive behavior greater than that of similarly aged children that negatively affects functioning in two or more settings.	• Screen for Childhood Anxiety-Related Emotional Disorders (SCARED) – self-report • Self-report Child Behavior Checklist (CBCL) self-report or caregiver report • Barratt Impulsiveness Scale (BIS) – self-report • Conners' Parent Rating Scale – caregiver report • CBCL – self-report or caregiver report
Eating disorders	**Binge eating** – the consumption of an unambiguously large amount of food during a constrained period of time while experiencing loss of control over the food consumption. **Loss of control eating** – feelings of loss of control over an episode of eating without consumption of an unambiguously large amount of food.	• Child Eating Disorder Examination (ChEDE) – structured interview • Youth Eating Disorder Examination– Questionnaire (YEDE-Q) – self-report
Cognitive functioning	**Deficits in executive function** – difficulties engaging in goal-directed behavior and overriding automatic responses. **Poor academic achievement** – poor performance on academic tasks (e.g., arithmetic, spelling, reading comprehension).	• Behavioral Rating Inventory of Executive Functions (BRIEF) – self-report, or caregiver or teacher report • Woodcock-Johnson III – Tests of Achievement – test battery

Internalizing and Externalizing Emotional and Behavioral Disorders

Children and adolescents with overweight and obesity are at increased risk for internalizing problems such as anxiety and depression (Luppino et al., 2010; Merikangas, Mendola, Pastor, Reuben, & Cleary, 2012), which may be explained by deficits in emotion regulation underlying both the obesogenic and internalizing behaviors (Puder & Munsch, 2010). For example, consumption of energy-dense palatable foods may serve as a coping strategy to reduce negative affect among children lacking other coping strategies, which would suggest that the internalizing behaviors precede obesity. To address this possibility, research needs to focus on adopting longitudinal designs, which allow researchers to test whether one negative consequence precedes the other. For example, one large study of adolescents in Grades 7–12 found that initial depression was a unique predictor of obesity 1 year later; in contrast, initial obesity did not predict depression 1 year later (Goodman & Whitaker, 2002). Similar results were obtained in a meta-analysis that examined multiple studies of depression and obesity among adolescents (Luppino et al., 2010). Thus, it may be that internalizing behaviors, such as depressive symptoms, are an early marker for future obesity risk in youth. On the other hand, children with overweight and obesity are more likely to be stigmatized by their peers and to experience negative social interactions (e.g., teasing), which may exacerbate internalizing behaviors.

Children with overweight also have difficulty regulating overt behavior, which may manifest as impulsivity or attention-deficit/hyperactivity disorder (ADHD) (Puder & Munsch, 2010). For example, researchers have documented a higher prevalence of ADHD in children with overweight and obesity in comparison with their peers with healthy weights (Waring & Lapane, 2008). Importantly, this association appears to be specific to children who are not taking stimulant medications; in fact, children taking stimulant medications for ADHD tend to experience underweight (Waring & Lapane, 2008). Significant behavior problems (including internalizing and externalizing behaviors) reported by a caregiver have been linked to concurrent overweight in children and to increased risk of experiencing overweight 2 years later, independent of potential sociodemographic confounding variables (Lumeng, Gannon, Cabral, Frank, & Zuckerman, 2003). Others have found that girls who experience overweight over the first 4 years of elementary school (kindergarten to Grade 3) also show increases in teacher-reported externalizing behaviors, as well as decreases in self-control, interpersonal skills, and academic performance over that same period of time (Datar & Sturm, 2006).

Eating Pathology

Two key pathological eating behaviors that have been shown to be comorbid with childhood obesity are *binge eating* and *loss of control* (LOC) eating. The former refers to the consumption of an unambiguously large amount of food during a constrained period of time while experiencing LOC over the food consumption. The latter refers to experiencing an LOC without eating an unambiguously large amount of food (Wilfley, Vannucci, & White, 2010). Both binge eating and LOC eating develop in childhood and both tend to be more prevalent among children with overweight as compared with their peers without overweight or obesity. Moreover, children at risk of obesity (either because they or their parents have overweight) who report LOC eating have been shown to be at increased risk for excess weight gain in the future, which suggests that LOC eating and binge eating disorder are risk factors for developing obesity (Tanofsky-Kraff, Yanovski, et al., 2009).

Cognition and Academic Achievement

Additionally, obesity has been linked to poorer cognitive functioning, especially in the domain of executive functions (Liang, Matheson, Kaye, & Boutelle, 2014). Executive functions are those cognitive processes involved in goal-oriented behavior and are critical to numerous aspects of a child's life, particularly those related to socioemotional and cognitive development (Best, Miller, & Jones, 2009). Research has linked both physical inactivity (Booth et al., 2013) and poor dietary habits (Davidson, Kanoski, Walls, & Jarrard, 2005) to deficits in executive functions, independent of weight status, which likely contributes to the association between obesity and poor cognitive functioning. Perhaps because children with overweight and obesity have poorer cognition, childhood obesity has been linked to lower academic achievement (Gable et al., 2012) and to lower educational attainment, in developed countries like the US (Cohen, Rai, Rehkopf, & Abrams, 2013). Along the same lines, difficulties with externalizing and internalizing problems may contribute to poorer classroom behavior and academic achievement, and vice versa (see Box 1).

Box 1
Points to Consider Regarding Psychosocial Comorbidities

1. A correlation may reflect reciprocal connections. For many (if not all) of these associations, it is likely that the associations are reciprocal, meaning that obesity may contribute to poorer psychosocial functioning, and concurrently, poor psychosocial functioning may contribute to obesity. Children with obesity may be ostracized and teased by their peers, leading to a dearth of quality friendships and to a host of psychological problems including anxiety and depression. At the same time, children with depression may turn to highly palatable, energy-dense foods to cope with the depression. As another example, children with poor executive function demonstrate diminished impulse control, which may make it difficult to abstain from eating highly rewarding, energy-dense foods. Additionally, research suggests that a poor diet (containing excess fatty foods) and a sedentary lifestyle may have detrimental effects on the child's brain and cognitive functions, which may manifest as poor executive function.

2. Psychological comorbidities are interrelated. A related point is that many of the psychosocial comorbidities are interrelated (Gable et al., 2012). Thus, not only are there bidirectional relations between a particular psychological comorbidity and obesity, there are likely bidirectional relations between comorbidities. As an example, academic difficulties might arise from cognitive deficits, and to complicate matters, academic difficulties may lead a child to withdraw from academic experiences, further exacerbating cognitive deficits. Similarly, academic difficulties may arise from poor social functioning and isolation.

3. Increased obesity severity, increased comorbidity severity. The severity of the comorbidity often increases with the severity and persistence of the obesity. This points to a common theme that was introduced previously: For many of the immediate and future negative consequences of obesity, there is a dose–response relationship. Therefore, clinicians should be particularly concerned for children who present with severe obesity, as those children may require more intensive treatment.

1.7   Diagnostic Procedures and Documentation

1.7.1   BMI

BMI is the routine screening metric for estimation of body composition and identification of obesity. BMI requires accurate measurement of a child's height and weight and can be easily calculated in a clinical setting. However, a child following the normal growth curve will experience a natural increase in BMI, which makes tracking weight status during weight loss treatment challenging. To account for this variation in BMI across age ranges, scores are typically standardized to ensure meaningful comparisons by providing a measure of relative overweight rather than absolute overweight. Common measures of relative overweight are described below.

BMI, BMI percentile, BMI z score, percentage overweight, and waist size are measures of child weight

BMI Percentile
Because BMI in youth naturally varies with the child's age and sex, measured values are converted to *BMI percentiles* before a diagnosis of obesity is made. BMI percentiles allow for the comparison of child weight status across the age range and by sex, by using reference data for age and sex derived from CDC growth curves. Children with a BMI that falls at or above the 85th percentile and below the 95th percentile are classified as having overweight, and children that fall at or above the 95th percentile are classified as having obesity. Thus, percentile scores are a measure of relative overweight or the degree of overweight present relative to that of a sex- and age-matched population. BMI percentile scores have a truncated upper limit, with a large portion of the distribution skewed in this direction (> 99th percentile). Because of the upper bounds on the measure, percentile scores are not sensitive to change in the upper ranges, limiting its utility for tracking child weight change over time. A more sensitive measure is the criteria for extreme obesity, which is a BMI at or above 120% of the sex-specific 95th percentile on the CDC BMI-for-age growth charts (Ogden et al., 2016).

BMI *Z* Score
BMI z score (also known as BMI standard deviation score) is another measure of relative weight that accounts for the change in BMI that naturally occurs as children age. BMI *z* score is calculated as the number of standard deviation units above or below the median, and accounts for the population weight distribution by utilizing reference data for age and sex derived from CDC growth curves for the calculation. The *z* score is also limited in that variability is reduced in the upper weight range (Berkey & Colditz, 2007).

Percentage Overweight
Percentage overweight is a measure of child relative weight and is calculated using a simple formula: 100×(child's BMI/50th percentile BMI for child's age and sex). Percentage overweight is sensitive to change throughout the entire BMI range and therefore may provide a more accurate estimation of obesity in children at the extreme end of the spectrum – that is, over the 99th percentile. Percentage overweight is not routinely used in clinical practice, but more often in research.

1.7.2   Waist Circumference

Waist circumference measurement is not routinely performed because it is not considered to provide additional information over BMI. The current expert committee recommendations for the prevention, assessment, and treatment of childhood obesity do not recommend waist circumference for clinical use, due to the lack of defined cutoffs (Spear et al., 2007). However, waist circumference may be a meaningful assessment tool for the estimation of abdominal obesity, the metabolically active fat associated with increased risk for cardiovascular disease and diabetes, and it may serve to identify children at greater risk of developing cardiovascular disease and diabetes (Gishti et al., 2015). Waist circumference has been associated with cardiovascular disease risk factors in both children (Maffeis, Pietrobelli, Grezzani, Provera, & Tato, 2001) and adolescents (Messiah, Arheart, Lipshultz, & Miller, 2008).

Waist circumference can be determined by a trained technician using a tape measure; accuracy can be increased by using a spring-loaded Gulick Tape Measure. A widely used protocol developed by NHANES described in the *Anthropometry Procedures Manual* (NHANES, 2011) measures the waist immediately above the right iliac crest at the midaxillary line. The WHO method measures the waist midway between the lowest rib margin and the iliac crest at the midaxillary line. Both methods are similar in ease of assessment of obesity and reproducibility. Despite the simplicity of the assessment, both intra- and inter-rater variabilities exist, especially in children with greater obesity. Waist circumference percentile estimates for children aged 2–18, by ethnicity, were developed in 2011 (Messiah, Arheart, Lipshultz, & Miller, 2011) identifying children at or above the 90th percentile at the greatest risk. Clinicians may consider assessing children for both BMI and waist circumference to capture a more complete overview of adiposity.

2

Theories and Models of the Disorder

2.1   Contributions of Child Eating Behavior to Obesity

2.1.1   Sugar-Sweetened Beverages

Sugar-sweetened beverages (SSBs), which include nondiet sodas, sweetened fruit juices and waters, sports and energy drinks, and sweetened coffees and teas have been implicated in the obesity epidemic and have become a target of public health campaigns designed to promote healthy weight development. The US Department of Health and Human Services and the US Department of Agriculture's *Dietary Guidelines for Americans* recommend reducing intake of SSBs because they provide little to no nutritional value and are a source of added sugars in the diet (US Department of Health and Human Services & US Department of Agriculture, 2015). Children who drink SSBs report higher daily energy intake than children who do not drink SSBs. Liquid calories possibly contribute to excess energy intake because beverages are quickly digested with minimal impact on satiety, therefore, individuals fail to compensate for this added energy by reducing food intake. Although soda consumption has declined in recent years, it is still the primary SSB consumed by youths in the US, with current estimates indicating children drink approximately 150–170 kilocalories of an SSB per day – the equivalent of one 12-oz (355-mL) beverage (Kit, Fakhouri, Park, Nielsen, & Ogden, 2013).

Research regarding the association between SSB consumption and weight gain is abundant, and while results generally support a positive relationship, discrepancies in findings have called a causal link into question. Early studies suggesting a positive relationship between SSB intake and weight gain in children were observational in nature, and over the last decade, several experimental trials have been conducted to test the relationship between SSBs and weight gain. For example, de Ruyter, Olthof, Seidell, & Katan (2012) conducted an 18-month randomized controlled trial of 641, 4- to 11-year-olds who were randomized to receive either an artificially sweetened, noncarbonated beverage, or a sugar-containing noncarbonated beverage. Children consumed one 250-mL can of the custom-designed beverage per day for the duration of the study. Results showed that children in the SSB group had significantly greater increases in BMI *z* score, weight, skinfold thickness, waist to height ratio, and fat mass than children in the artificially sweetened beverage group. Ebbeling and colleagues implemented an intervention to reduce SSB consumption in 224 adolescents (Ebbeling et al., 2012). Results at 1 year showed a significantly smaller increase in BMI for adolescents in the intervention group compared

SSB consumption in children leads to greater daily energy intakes

SSBs have been implicated in the obesity epidemic

with those in the control group. However, this difference was not evident at the 2-year follow-up. The preliminary data from these experimental trials support a causal link between SSB consumption and weight; however, more research is needed. Despite the lack of conclusive evidence for a causal relationship between SSBs and weight gain, recommendations to limit children's consumption of these beverages are still warranted because SSBs are a source of added energy and provide no nutritional benefits.

2.1.2   Food Away From Home

High intake of FAFH has been associated with child obesity

Many families are choosing to eat out rather than prepare home-cooked meals. For example, only half of American households currently report cooking dinner at home (Virudachalam, Long, Harhay, Polsky, & Feudtner, 2014). It comes as no surprise then that children and adolescents consume approximately one third of their energy from *food away from home* (FAFH), with adolescents consuming the greatest proportion (37%) (Poti & Popkin, 2011). Rates of FAFH in populations with high overweight and obesity may be even higher (Altman et al., 2015). The trend toward increased consumption of foods prepared outside the home coincides with the increased rates of childhood obesity and has been implicated as a primary contributor to this epidemic. Consumption of FAFH has been shown to lead to weight gain in children and adolescents over time (Fulkerson et al., 2011). Even consuming as little as one meal per week away from home increases a child's risk for obesity (Ayala et al., 2008).

FAHF is higher in calories and fat, with larger portion sizes

FAFH generally contains more energy, fat, and sodium, and fewer healthful nutrients such as fiber, calcium, and iron, than food prepared at home (Guthrie, Lin, & Frazao, 2002), and portion sizes are typically larger (Young & Nestle, 2002), resulting in excess energy intake (Piernas & Popkin, 2011). Powell and Nguyen (2013) reported that FAFH consumption was associated with a net increase of 160.5 and 267.3 kcal in children and adolescents, respectively. Frequent dining out also detracts from the overall quality of the diet and the food environment of the home. In children, FAFH consumption is positively associated with fat, added sugars, and SSBs, and negatively associated with fiber, milk, fruits, and nonstarchy vegetables (Bowman, Gortmaker, Ebbeling, Pereira, & Ludwig, 2004; Powell & Nguyen, 2013). FAFH frequency is also associated with having more soda and chips in the home and serving fewer healthy foods at home such as vegetables and milk (Boutelle, Cafri, & Crow, 2012). Preliminary data suggest that reducing FAFH may be an important target for weight loss by improving the overall quality of the diet. Altman et al. (2015) examined FAFH in 241 children who participated in a weight loss trial and found that children who reduced their FAFH lost the most weight. The reported association was mediated by an increase in diet quality.

Multiple barriers to the consumption of foods prepared at home have been reported in the literature. With more women in the labor force, more children are being raised in households with two parents working outside the home, which leaves fewer daily hours available for household management tasks such as meal planning and preparation (Archer et al., 2013). In fact, time spent in the kitchen has decreased significantly since the 1960s (Jabs & Devine 2006). Scarcity of time, inadequate cooking skills, and the lack of kitchen supplies have been reported as obstacles to meal preparation at home (Appelhans, Waring, Schneider, & Pagoto, 2014; Fulkerson et al., 2011). In addition to these constraints, parents also cite the challenge of trying to please a variety of individual taste preferences and dealing with the limited diets of picky eaters, as barriers when cooking meals at home (Fulkerson et al., 2011). Given these challenges, many families choose not to eat at home or choose not to cook at home given the increased availability and convenience of prepared foods. Support for families in meal planning and preparation is needed to address these barriers and reduce the frequency of eating away from home.

2.1.3   Breakfast

Breakfast is defined as the meal that is consumed within 2–3 hrs of waking, includes at least one food group, and contributes 15–25% of daily energy intake (O'Neil et al., 2014). A healthy breakfast is defined as one that includes at least 3 food groups and improves overall daily nutrient intake. The ideal breakfast includes protein-rich foods coupled with nutrient-dense, carbohydrate-rich grains, fruits, or vegetables. A sample of healthy breakfast choices can be seen in Box 2. Even though breakfast has long been recognized as the most important meal of the day, a concept now supported by a wide array of scientific evidence, approximately 20% of children and 30% of adolescents report skipping it (Deshmukh-Taskar et al., 2010). Reported barriers to breakfast consumption in youths include the absence of hunger, time constraints, and lack of planning.

Breakfast is recognized as most important meal of the day

Eating breakfast is associated with healthy body weight and lifestyle behaviors

Many adolescents report skipping meals as a form of dieting to lose weight; however, following a healthful eating pattern that includes a quality breakfast is recommended for the promotion of weight management and improved dietary intake (US Department of Health and Human Services & US Department of Agriculture, 2015). Breakfast consumption in youths is associated with better overall diet quality and more favorable nutrient intake (Matthys, De Henauw, Bellemans, De Maeyer, & De Backer, 2007). Breakfast consumers are more likely to have a healthy body weight and engage in healthier lifestyle behaviors such as exercise (Widenhorn-Muller, Hille, Klenk, & Weiland, 2008). Eating breakfast may also be beneficial for the prevention of chronic disease, as breakfast consumption in childhood (Smith et al., 2010) and adolescence (Wennberg, Gustafsson, Wennberg, & Hammarstrom, 2015) has been shown to be protective against the future development of heart disease, diabetes, and obesity. Breakfast consumption may also improve cognitive function, as studies have shown that children who eat breakfast report greater concentration and higher academic performance than breakfast skippers (Widenhorn-Muller et al., 2008).

Box 2
Healthy Breakfast Options and Suggestions for Increasing Breakfast Consumption

Breakfast definitions:

The first meal of the day consumed within 2–3 hrs of waking. May be consumed at any location and includes at least one food group and contributes 15–25% of daily energy intake. A healthy breakfast is defined as including at least three food groups, such as protein-rich foods coupled with nutrient-dense, carbohydrate-rich grains, fruits, or vegetables.

Examples of healthy breakfasts:

1. One fruit and cereal bar, 1 oz of string cheese, one medium-size banana;
2. One cup shredded wheat cereal, one cup fat-free milk, one-half cup strawberries;
3. One scrambled egg, one tablespoon low-fat, shredded cheddar cheese, one orange, one slice wheat toast with two teaspoons 100% fruit spread;
4. Three-quarter cup nonfat blueberry yogurt, one-half whole grain bagel, one tablespoon low-fat cream cheese, one orange;
5. One slice whole wheat toast, one tablespoon peanut butter, one medium banana, one apple;
6. One English muffin, one fried egg, 1 oz Canadian bacon, one cup fat-free milk, one cup melon cubes;
7. One whole grain waffle, one tablespoon maple syrup, one cup fat-free fruit yogurt, one-half cup blueberries;

Strategies for increasing frequency of breakfast consumption:

1. Educate families on the importance of breakfast for health and academic performance;
2. Encourage families to plan ahead;
   a. Organize refrigerated breakfast foods for easy access;
   b. The night before
      i. Set out tableware and nonperishable foods;
      ii. Wash and cut fresh fruit, hard boil eggs, blend yogurt and fresh fruit for a smoothie, etc.;
   c. Have already prepared foods available for a quick on-the-go meal when in a rush (e.g., trail mix, dried fruit, fiber-rich cereal bars);
3. Encourage parents to model eating breakfast for their children by eating together;
4. Help families on limited budgets identify food assistance programs such as the School Breakfast Program, Supplemental Nutrition Assistance Program, and the Special Supplemental Nutrition Assistance Program for Women, Infants, and Children.

Note. Based on O'Neil et al., 2014

The mechanisms behind the weight-related effects of breakfast are not completely understood. Current research suggests that consumption of a meal after the overnight fast affects appetite and energy balance through metabolic changes in blood glucose, insulin regulation, and lipid metabolism (Pereira et al., 2011). The composition of breakfast may also influence weight by affecting these physiological variables, with a higher protein meal providing preferred effects. Leidy, Hoertel, Douglas, Higgins, and Shafer (2015) conducted an intervention to promote breakfast consumption in adolescents with overweight or obesity who were regular breakfast skippers. They found that adolescents who were instructed to consume a high-protein breakfast (35 g protein) reported less daily hunger and greater reductions in daily calorie intake than those adolescents who continued to skip breakfast. Further fat mass gain was prevented in the high-protein breakfast group over the course of the 12-week intervention.

Breakfast consumption is an important health behavior, with benefits that extend beyond weight management. Families receiving weight loss treatment should be informed of the benefits of a healthy breakfast and provided with strategies to address common barriers to breakfast consumption.

Breakfast is an important health behavior, with benefits that extend beyond weight management

2.2   Contributions of Child Physical Inactivity and Sedentary Behaviors to Obesity

Increased rates of sedentary behaviors and decreased participation in physical activities in children and adolescents may also be primary contributors to the high rates of childhood obesity. More than half of 9- to 13-year-olds do not participate in any organized physical activities (CDC, 2003; Cooper et al., 2015). The American Academy of Pediatrics (AAP) recommends that entertainment screen time should be limited to less than 1–2 hrs per day for children 2–18 years old (Council on Sports Medicine and Fitness & Council on School Health, 2006). The American Heart Association recommends that all children aged 2 and older should participate in at least 60 min of enjoyable, moderate to vigorous physical activities every day that are developmentally appropriate and varied. See Table 6 for a summary of recommendations for different age groups.

The AAP recommends limiting children's entertainment screen time < 1–2 hrs/day

2.3   Role of Appetitive Traits in Childhood Obesity

In the context of childhood obesity, *appetitive traits* refer to stable behavioral phenotypes related to dysregulated eating and food consumption that promote a positive energy balance (Wilfley et al., 2010). Key among these are impulsivity (mentioned previously in Section 1.6.2 "Psychosocial Comorbidities"), satiety responsiveness, and a motivation to consume palatable foods (van den Berg et al., 2011). Research suggests that these traits may be heritable, likely due to shared genetic and environmental factors between parents and children that influence the development and maintenance of these appetitive traits (Epstein, Paluch, Beecher, & Roemmich, 2008).

Appetitive traits are stable behavioral patterns associated with food consumption

Table 6
Recommendations for Physical Activity in Children From the American Academy of Pediatrics

Age group	Recommendations
Infants and toddlers	• No television for children under the age of 2 years • Allowed to develop enjoyment of outdoor physical activity and unstructured exploration with responsible adult caregiver (i.e., walking or unorganized free play outdoors)
Preschool (4–6 years old)	• Limit screen time to < 2 hrs per day • Free play should be encouraged with emphasis on fun, playfulness, and exploration (i.e., running, swimming, tumbling, throwing, catching)
Elementary School (6–9 years old)	• Free play should continue to be encouraged, involving more sophisticated movement patterns with emphasis on fundamental skill acquisition (walk, dance, jump rope) • Organized sports should have flexible rules and short instruction time • Allow free time in practices and focus on enjoyment rather than competition • Co-ed participation is not contraindicated, as few differences between sexes exists
Middle School (10–12 years)	• Preferred physical activities that focus on enjoyment should be encouraged • Skill development and factors that promote continued participation are needed • Placement for contact and collusion sports should be based on maturity rather than chronological age • Weight training may be initiated, with low weight and high repetitions
Adolescents	• Identify activities that are of interest and fun, and include friends • Enrollment in competitive sports should be based on size and ability rather than chronological age

Based on Council on Sports Medicine and Fitness & Council on School Health, 2006. Available at http://pediatrics.aappublications.org/content/pediatrics/117/5/1834.full.pdf

2.3.1   Impulsivity

The concept of impulsivity was mentioned briefly in the context of externalizing behavior (Section 1.6.2 "Psychosocial Comorbidities"). Here its specific role in controlling appetitive behavior is discussed. Impulsivity refers to a diminished ability to resist immediate temptations that stand in conflict with future outcomes or long-term goals. For example, for a child in a weight management program, choosing to eat a piece of cake may be conceptualized as an impulsive behavior because it conflicts with a long-term goal (i.e., lose excess weight). Impulsivity can be assessed in a variety of ways in children, including via parent- and teacher-reported measures and behavioral assessment. One classic behavioral assessment is the *marshmallow task* (Mischel, Shoda, & Rodriguez, 1989), in which an experimenter presents a child with a marshmallow and states that if the child can wait for a period of time (e.g., 5–10 min) then the child will receive two marshmallows. During the interim, the experimenter states that she needs to leave the room and if the child cannot wait until she returns, the child can notify the experimenter (e.g., with a bell) and have the single marshmallow immediately. This task, as well as variations using other food and nonfood rewards, has been employed in children as young as age 3, and it has been used to demonstrate that children with a diminished ability to delay gratification are heavier at the time of the experiment and at risk of gaining excess weight in later childhood or adolescence (Francis & Susman, 2009). Remarkably, young children with high impulsivity as measured by this task were found to be heavier even 30 years later as adults, even after adjusting for other important factors (Schlam, Wilson, Shoda, Mischel, & Ayduk, 2013). Although the marshmallow task may provide a direct assessment of impulsivity, it may not be feasible for use in clinical practice due to time and other constraints. As such, parent-reported measures may be valuable – for example, the Behavioral Rating Inventory of Executive Functions (Gioia, Isquith, Guy, & Kenworthy, 2000) is able to capture several cognitive functions related to impulsivity (e.g., inhibitory control). Additionally, self-report measures, such as the commonly used Barratt Impulsiveness Scale (Patton, Stanford, & Barratt, 1995), have been used with children as young as 10 (Steinberg et al., 2009).

2.3.2   Motivation to Consume Palatable Food

The *motivation to consume palatable foods* refers to how much work one is willing to do to obtain a certain food. In general, people are motivated to eat food because it is necessary for survival; however, this motivation varies across individuals, contexts, and foods. Research suggests that heavier children have higher motivation to consume palatable foods compared with their leaner peers (Temple, Legierski, Giacomelli, Salvy, & Epstein, 2008), and children with high motivation to consume palatable foods are at greater risk of gaining excess weight (Hill, Saxton, Webber, Blundell, & Wardle, 2009). A child's motivation to consume palatable foods can be assessed using the relative reinforcing value of food (RRVfood) task (Temple et al., 2008). In this task, children are asked to make choices between receiving a certain palatable food and an alternative reward (e.g., 5 min of free play). Over time, the work associated with making the food choice increases relative to the alternative (e.g., at first, the child may need to press a button five times to receive the food reward or the 5 min of free play, but later 50 button presses are required for food). A child with a high motivation to consume palatable foods will work harder for the food reward, whereas a child with a lower motivation will decide earlier on to choose the alternative because it requires less work. A questionnaire version of this behavioral task has been developed and validated in adults (Goldfield, Epstein, Davidson, & Saad, 2005), which has also been shown to have predictive validity in children (Best et al., 2012; Hill et al., 2009).

2.3.3   Satiety Responsiveness

Satiety responsiveness refers to one's ability to perceive and respond to internal cues of fullness. It can be assessed in the laboratory by measuring a child's consumption of palatable food after having eaten a meal (i.e., eating in the absence of hunger; Wardle, Guthrie, Sanderson, & Rapoport, 2001). Children who eat more in these laboratory conditions are said to have poor satiety responsiveness (i.e., difficulties recognizing and properly responding to cues signaling satiety). This method for assessing satiety responsiveness may not be feasible in a clinical practice (Wilfley et al., 2010). Therefore, an alternative is the Child Eating Behavior Questionnaire (CEBQ), which contains a satiety responsiveness subscale. This instrument takes only a brief period of time to complete, and the respondent is the parent or caregiver (Wardle et al., 2001). Research has shown that this measure explains a significant amount of the variance in observed eating behavior in young children, thus supporting its validity (Carnell & Wardle, 2007). Moreover, satiety responsive, as measured by the CEBQ, is associated with increased relative weight and waist circumference in children (Carnell & Wardle, 2008).

Appetitive traits may impact a child's ability to make positive behavioral changes

Children with combinations of these appetitive traits may be at even greater risk for obesity compared with children with only one of these traits. Moreover, children with overweight and obesity with multiple appetitive traits may be more resistant to standard weight loss treatments compared with children with fewer appetitive traits. For example, children with high impulsivity coupled with a high motivation to consume palatable snack foods showed poorer weight loss during a 16-week family-based behavioral weight loss treatment (FBT), compared with children with only high impulsivity or high motivation for such foods (Best et al., 2012). Because of the important role of these appetitive traits in obesity and its treatment, current research is examining ways to reduce impulsivity and food-related motivation. This line of research includes targeted training of the neurocognitive processes related to restraining impulsive behavior (Houben & Jansen, 2011) and training individuals to bias their thinking toward future events, rather than immediate ones (Daniel, Stanton, & Epstein, 2013).

2.4   Behavioral Economics and Obesity

Behavioral economics involves understanding how people makes choices

One way to understand the determinants of obesity is to apply the study of how and why people make choices, termed *behavioral economics* (Epstein, Salvy, Carr, Dearing, & Bickel, 2010). Behavioral economics is a melding of economic and psychological principles, and can be used by clinicians to understand the environmental and psychological factors that may lead people to make healthy or unhealthy choices (see Box 3). As such, behavioral economics does not deal strictly with the child's behavior, but looks at how the child's behavior may be influenced by certain environmental conditions. A key idea in behavioral economics is that two behaviors can be complements of one another, substitutes for one another, or they can be completely unrelated. For example, eating popcorn and watching a movie are often complementary activities. In contrast, jogging at a brisk pace and eating popcorn are substituting behaviors. If people are engaging in vigorous activity, such as jogging, they are not likely to also be eating popcorn. Substitutes and complements indirectly influence the frequency of one another. For example, if the home is set up to encourage television watching (e.g., there are TVs in most rooms, there is a big screen television with surround sound stereo), this may also encourage unhealthy snacking behavior because watching TV and snacking often occur concurrently. If, on the other hand, the home is set up to encourage physical activity (e.g., by providing recreational equipment, parental support for physical activity), this may reduce snacking because the two activities do not go together.

Setting up the home to provide substitutes for snacking can reduce excess eating

Box 3
Behavioral Economic Concepts

Behavioral economics departs from classical economic theory by exploring the ways in which people make decisions that are irrational (i.e., decisions that do not maximize gains while minimizing losses). It has interesting applications, including to increase our understanding of the behavioral choices that result in energy imbalances related to obesity. Some key definitions of behavioral economic concepts that may help explicate obesogenic behaviors are:

Substitutes: behaviors or commodities that replace one another – that is, engaging in one behavior (or obtaining one commodity) *decreases* the likelihood of engaging in the other behavior (or buying the other commodity). Drinking SSBs may substitute for drinking water or milk.

Complements: behaviors or commodities that go hand-in-hand – that is, engaging in one behavior (or obtaining one commodity) *increases* the likelihood of engaging in the other behavior (or buying the other commodity). Watching television is a complement for snacking.

Opportunity costs: activities (or commodities) forfeited in the process of engaging in an alternative activity (or purchasing an alternative commodity). For example, if a child spends her free time after school going to swim practice, that free time cannot be used to play video games.

Delay discounting: rewards received in the future are not worth as much to us as immediate rewards. For example, if given the option of having $10 today or $12 in 2 years, many people would rather have the $10 today because they discount $12 as a function of the delay to its receipt (2 years). Children may discount delayed rewards associated with healthy behavior (e.g., improved cardiovascular health as adults) and therefore choose activities with immediate rewards (e.g., eating a cupcake provides an immediate feeling of pleasure) but with longer-term negative consequences in the form of excessive weight gain.

Another important behavioral economic concept is opportunity cost. Opportunity cost refers to the alternative activity(ies) given up in the process of choosing a particular activity (Finkelstein & Strombotne, 2010). For example, if a child engages in physical activity, the opportunity cost could be time spent playing a highly enjoyable video game. The greater the number or severity of opportunity costs, the greater the barriers to engaging in a desired health behavior. Clinicians should be aware of potential opportunity costs and work with families to minimize these. If time allotted to television watching or video game playing is restricted, this may result in physical activity being a compelling alternative because the opportunity costs have been reduced. A complementary approach is to work with the family to identify physical activities that are highly reinforcing for the child and strategize how these can become more easily available to the child. Together, by decreasing barriers to desired physical activity and increasing barriers to undesired activities, the likelihood that the child will engage in physical activity should increase.

2.5   Family Influences on Weight

Children are more likely to develop obesity if their parents have obesity

It is not surprising that the family exerts influence over a child's behavior, including those behaviors related to eating and physical activity. While the magnitude of this influence has been debated, the current consensus is that the family influence over the child's eating and activity behaviors – and in turn, the child's weight status – is significant. For example, one study determined that toddlers (1–2 years old) with one parent with obesity were 3.2 times more likely to have obesity in young adulthood (21–29 years old) compared with toddlers with parents with normal weight, and toddlers with two parents with obesity were 13.6 times more likely to have obesity (Whitaker, Wright, Pepe, Seidel, & Dietz, 1997).

Interestingly, the toddler's own weight status was not a predictor of their future risk for obesity. A study supporting this finding used a statistical technique called *receiver operating characteristic* (ROC) *curve analysis* (Morandi et al., 2012). This type of analysis is used frequently in medicine to evaluate whether a diagnostic test can correctly identify whether an individual has a specific condition or disease (a *true positive*) but avoid incorrectly concluding a disease or condition is present (a *false positive*). Specifically, test accuracy is evaluated by examining the area under the ROC curve. If the area under the curve is 1.0, the test is perfect; if it is 0.5, it does no better than chance and is therefore uninformative. In this particular study of parental influences on offspring obesity, paternal and maternal BMI were the best predictors of whether a newborn came to have obesity in later childhood or adolescence. Knowledge of both parents' BMI boosted the area under the ROC curve from 0.5 to approximately 0.65–0.72, depending on when obesity was assessed. The inclusion of additional factors related to the family, including gestational weight gain, maternal smoking, and number of members in the household, improved the area under the ROC curve a bit more, such that the final area ranged from 0.67–0.75. Thus, although knowledge of these familial factors does not make a perfect diagnostic tool, it does help the clinician determine whether a child is at elevated risk for overweight or obesity.

Knowledge of both parents' BMI is important in assessing obesity risk in children

Effective prevention and treatment must include family members as well as the at-risk child

Table 7 lists some of the ways in which obesity may be transmitted via behavioral mechanisms from parent to offspring. These influences involve both the shaping of the physical home environment (e.g., by purchasing certain foods or by purchasing certain goods that encourage physical activity vs. inactivity) and the shaping of the psychological and behavioral environment of the home (e.g., by modeling or encouraging certain behaviors). Therefore, effective prevention and treatment of childhood obesity must deal with family members in addition to the at-risk child. The greater the magnitude of positive behavior change made by the surrounding family members (e.g., caregivers, siblings, and even grandparents), the greater the child's likelihood for successful weight loss.

Table 7
Parental Influences on Children's Eating and Activity Behaviors

Type of influence	Source of parental influence	Potential effects of parental influence
Parental influences on the physical home environment	Parent purchases food for the home, determines meal times and eating routine, and prepares the food	*Negative sources of influence* • Fresh fruits and vegetables are not purchased, resulting in limited access to these foods • Meals may be served infrequently or erratically, prompting snacking between meals *Positive sources of influence* • Parents purchase fresh fruits, vegetables, and lean meats and few packaged or "junk" foods • Family meals are eaten at home at relatively regular times, and snacks are planned
	Parents determine how the home is equipped and set household rules and routines	*Negative sources of influence* • Parents may allow for televisions and video gaming equipment in multiple rooms, including bedrooms, which encourages inactivity and may disrupt sleep • Watching television or playing video games also complements snacking and can increase energy intake by disrupting habituation to food and satiety *Positive sources of influence* • Parents have a designated area and times for screen-based activities (e.g., the den) • Parents purchase recreational equipment that the family would enjoy using together; keeping this equipment accessible and in good working order
Parental behavioral influences	Parental modeling of lifestyle behaviors and associative learning	*Negative sources of influence* • Children view their parents' unhealthy eating and activity behaviors and adopt these behaviors as their own • Family routines or habits that pair food with certain events cause children to associate certain foods with these events or activities (e.g., "It's Friday night, so we're going to have pizza" becomes "It's Friday night, so we must have pizza") *Positive sources of influence* • Parents engage in healthy eating during family meals and participate in physical activities that their child can do as well • Activities that do not involve food are planned that the family can enjoy together ("It's Saturday afternoon, so we're going on a hike")

Table7 (continued)

Parental behavioral influences	Parenting practices encourage or restrict a child's behaviors	*Negative sources of influence* • A parent's restrictive feeding practices may lead to a child's preoccupation with, and stronger preference for, the restricted food • A parent's frequent prompts to their child to "eat up" may encourage faster rates of eating • A parent's use of food as a reward may increase a child's preference for the food that is used as a reward, even if that food is used to encourage a child to consume a healthy food (e.g., "If you eat your broccoli, you can have dessert"; the child will come to prefer dessert, not the broccoli) *Positive sources of influence* • A parent engineers the home so that access to healthy, palatable foods is increased, and unhealthy foods are not available so the parent does not need to use restriction to decrease a child's intake of unhealthy foods (e.g., "You can have an apple or grapes for your snack" – because these are the only snack foods available – instead of, "Don't eat the chips for your snack")

2.6   Environmental Influences on Weight

Dramatic changes in environment have had an impact on increases in childhood obesity

Until 30 or 40 years ago, obesity rates were stable and low in the US and elsewhere, but since then, they have nearly tripled. Given the slow rate at which genes change in a population, the likely causes for this rapid increase in the rates of obesity are the dramatic and swift changes in the environment that surrounds us. This is not to say that genetics are not important to obesity (see next section), but only that genetic changes have not been a major contributor to the increases in obesity over the past 3–4 decades. Instead, there have been many changes to the environment across contexts, from the food environment (e.g., the types of foods available in the school cafeteria or the supermarket) to the built environment (e.g., infrastructure and buildings that surround us) to the school curricula (e.g., the amount of time in the school day dedicated to physical education and recess), which correlate with increases in obesity. Box 4 provides an overview of some these influences on eating behavior and physical activity.

The built environment refers to the infrastructure and buildings around us

Box 4
Environmental Changes That Influence Childhood Obesity

Food intake	• The price of fresh fruits and vegetables has increased at a greater rate than the price of fats, oils, and sugar-sweetened beverages
	• Portion sizes have increased substantially, contributing to overeating
	• Technology allows for easy and quick preparation of foods that are typically energy-dense yet nutrient-poor (e.g., microwaveable meals)
	• Cheap and easy-to-prepare foods increase the likelihood of snacking between meals
Physical activity	• Ownership of personal cars has increased, reducing the need for active forms of transportation (e.g., cycling, walking)
	• Changes in the built environment (e.g., highways rather than walkable boulevards) have decreased the safety of walking or cycling
	• Mandatory physical education in the schools has been reduced, leading to decreased opportunities for physical activity during the school day
	• The number and scope of "passive" leisure-time activities have increased (e.g., interactive video games, cable television with hundreds of channels), dissuading children from engaging in physical activity during their free time

These dramatic changes to the food and built environments, and their associated negative consequences, have prompted some to suggest that government intervention is needed to help curb childhood obesity (Finkelstein & Strombotne, 2010). These interventions could involve the government's reconsideration of certain food subsidies that promote the availability and consumption of highly processed foods and SSBs by lowering their prices or incentivizing their production. Also, the government could provide the infrastructure and support for transportation projects that would increase pedestrian safety and provide bicycle lanes. A now famous (and contentious) example of a governmental intervention at the policy level within the US is Mayor Michael Bloomberg's attempt to ban large sugary drinks in New York City.

Although clinicians may have little influence on the broader food and built environments that surround a family struggling with overweight and obesity, the clinician should be aware of these influences and should work with families to create strategies to deal with these environmental influences. For example, clinicians can help families recognize and make use of positive environmental factors (e.g., proximate parks and other recreational facilities) while avoiding negative influences (e.g., dining out should be limited due to large portion sizes and energy-dense ingredients).

Families can become aware of how the larger environment impacts energy intake and expenditure

2.7   Genetic Influences

As mentioned above, our individual genetics do not provide a good explanation for why childhood obesity has reached epidemic proportions in recent decades, but our genes can help explain why some children are more prone to obesity than others. Heritability studies (i.e., studies that compare characteristics of identical twins reared together vs. apart) suggest that approximately 50% of the variance in BMI is genetic in origin (Allison et al., 1996). Compared with estimates of the heritability of height (approximately 80%; Yang et al., 2010), genes play an important – but not decisive – role in the differences in obesity across individuals.

Studies of large numbers of participants (numbering in the thousands, if not tens of thousands) that have looked across the human genome have identified several genes that consistently correlate with variation in BMI (Speliotes et al., 2010). The most commonly examined obesity gene is the fat mass and obesity-associated (FTO) gene. Its precise function is largely unknown; however, recent research suggests that FTO gene plays a larger role in peripheral metabolism (i.e., the conversion of food into energy) than it does in central neuronal regulation of metabolism (McMurray et al., 2013). In children, it has been shown that individuals with high-risk FTO alleles (i.e., FTO alleles associated with increased BMI) eat more food in a laboratory setting (Wardle, Llewellyn, Sanderson, & Plomin, 2009) and report more eating episodes with LOC (Tanofsky-Kraff, Han, et al., 2009). See Table 8 for more information about some of these common genes, including the FTO gene.

Table 8
Common Gene Variants Associated With Obesity in Children and Adults

Gene	Frequency of obesity-increasing allele	Function
Fat mass and obesity-associated (FTO) gene	0.42	Peripheral metabolic functioning
Melanocortin 4 receptor (MC4R) gene	0.24	Neuronal regulation of appetite or energy balance
Brain-derived neurotrophic factor (BDNF) gene	0.78	Neuronal regulation of appetite or energy balance
Pro-opiomelanocortin (POMC) gene	0.47	Neuronal regulation of appetite or energy balance
Gastric inhibitory polypeptide receptor (GIPR) gene	0.80	Peripheral metabolic functioning
SH2B1 gene	0.40	Neuronal regulation of appetite or energy balance

Note. Based on Coll & Loraine Tung, 2009; Huszar et al., 1997; Li, Zhou, Carter-Su, Myers, & Rui, 2007; McMurray et al., 2013; Ren et al., 2007; Saxena et al., 2010; Unger, Calderon, Bradley, Sena-Esteves, & Rios, 2007

However, a perplexing finding is that together these known genes account for at most 2% of the variation in BMI, which is in stark contrast to the 50% heritability estimate mentioned above. This issue of "missing heritability" is a major challenge in the field of behavioral genetics. It is likely that rare gene variants and numerous other genes that account for very small proportions of variance alone are responsible for some of this discrepancy between the 2% and 50% estimates (Llewellyn, Trzaskowski, Plomin, & Wardle, 2013). Moreover, there may be interactive effects among genes, such that the combined effects are not simply the addition of each gene's individual effects on obesity risk.

For clinicians, an important question is how genes factor into assessing the risk for future obesity in children and/or help in prescribing treatment. Regarding the assessment of risk, a recent study suggests that genes are a significant predictor of newborns' future risk for obesity, but this effect is greatly overshadowed by the effects of parental weight status (Morandi et al., 2012) – that is, the best predictor of a newborn's risk for obesity in the future is whether that newborn's parents have obesity. This risk is partially due to shared genes, but also to parenting behavior related to eating and activity that affects the weight of both the parent and the child. As will be discussed in Chapter 4, this suggests that treatments of childhood obesity should include parents in order to have the largest, and most sustainable, effects on weight (Wilfley et al., 2010). This finding also suggests that clinicians should be aware of parental BMI when assessing obesity risk in children and youths. Moreover, assessing parental height and weight to calculate BMI is more cost effective than conducting genetic testing.

Treatments of childhood obesity should include the parents

It is currently unclear what role genes play in obesity treatment outcomes. For example, some studies have found that the FTO gene impacts participants' weight loss response to certain dietary interventions (e.g., Zhang et al., 2012), but other studies have not found this (e.g., Franks et al., 2008). Thus, while this is an active area of research and future breakthroughs are likely, the evidence so far does not indicate a clear role for genetics in customizing behavioral treatments for children and families.

The role of genetics in obesity treatment is unclear

3

Diagnosis and Treatment Indications

3.1   Diagnosis

The recommended metric for determining whether a child has overweight or obesity is the BMI percentile specific to that child's age and sex (August et al., 2008; Barlow & Expert Committee, 2007). BMI does not measure body fat directly, but it is a feasible clinical assessment that correlates with body fat and cardiovascular risk. Current recommendations are that children whose BMI is > 85th percentile and < 95th percentile be categorized as having *overweight* and children whose BMI is ≥ 95th percentile be categorized as having *obesity*. For children at the ends of the developmental spectrum, BMI percentile may not be appropriate. For adolescents, obesity is defined as BMI ≥ 95th percentile or BMI ≥ 30 – whichever is lower. For children under the age of 2, weight-for-height values > 95th percentile for the child's age indicate overweight (Barlow & Expert Committee, 2007). Although BMI provides a rough estimate of a child's risk, it is recommended that the clinician, in concert with the primary care physician, gather additional information to get a clearer picture of the child's risk and to make recommendations regarding prevention and treatment. This additional information includes physiological comorbidities, the presence of obesity in other family members, the typical eating and activity patterns of the child, and the motivations, concerns, and confidence related to obesity and behavior change. Using this information, the clinician can make recommendations related to prevention and treatment, which will be discussed in detail in Chapter 4.

Height and weight are not the only information important to providing treatment recommendations

3.2   Treatment Predictors

Once it is determined that treatment is recommended, a detailed understanding of individual and familial factors that have been shown to be predictive of weight loss outcomes can help with the development of the most effective and tailored treatment for a child. These factors fall into one of two categories: *general predictors* explain why a child is successful or not, irrespective of the type of treatment provided, while *treatment-specific predictors* (also referred to as treatment moderators) identify whether a child will respond favorably to a specific type of treatment but not to another. Much of the research identifying these predictive factors is nascent – especially that evaluating treatment-specific predictors – and not all studies provide consistent findings; however, it is worth pointing out some of the predictive factors to keep in mind.

3.2.1   Demographic Factors

Younger children have been shown to be more successful than older children in weight control programs (Goldschmidt et al., 2014; Sabin et al., 2007; Yildirim et al., 2011), perhaps because obesogenic habits are less ingrained in younger children. Also, younger children still have a lot of height growth ahead of them, which means that they need to lose less weight to obtain a nonoverweight status as they continue to grow taller (Goldschmidt, Wilfley, Paluch, Roemmich, & Epstein, 2013). These findings highlight the need for early intervention, which may be more effective given both increased ease of altering behavior and the requirement for more modest weight loss to achieve nonoverweight status in younger children. However, these findings should not be taken to suggest that older children do not succeed in treatment. For example, one study showed that older children (≥ 10.3 years) achieved substantial weight loss followed by weight maintenance, in a family-based weight loss program that focused on increasing fruits and vegetables rather than on decreasing energy-dense foods (Epstein et al., 2008).

There is some question about whether boys or girls show better responses to family-based weight loss treatments (Best et al., 2012; Epstein, Paluch, & Raynor, 2001). In a study comparing two variations of family-based treatment, boys did equally well when the focus was on increasing fruits and vegetables or decreasing energy-dense foods, whereas girls did substantially better when the focus was on increasing fruits and vegetables (Epstein et al., 2008). In a meta-analysis of school-based interventions, the general conclusion across studies was that girls had better outcomes than boys in terms of changes in energy-balance behaviors (Yildirim et al., 2011).

Although racial and ethnic minority children – especially African American and Hispanic children – tend to be at greater risk for overweight and obesity, the evidence is not strong that they show poorer success in behavioral weight management treatments. In the meta-analysis of school-based interventions mentioned above, there was no consistent evidence that minority children did any better or worse in school-based interventions (Yildirim et al., 2011). Similarly, most studies of family-based interventions using ethnically diverse samples indicate that minority children do as well as their White counterparts, both at intervention completion and following a long-term follow-up (Goldschmidt et al., 2014; Savoye et al., 2011). We are aware of only one study in which ethnic and racial minority children (primarily African American and Hispanic children) lost less weight at the end of a 16-week family-based treatment (Best et al., 2012); however, unpublished data from this study showed that after more than one and a half years after the end of treatment, these racial and ethnic differences were no longer significant.

3.2.2   Family Factors

There is a negative correlation between parent weight and child weight loss success, such that children of heavier parents show poorer treatment success (Goldschmidt et al., 2014; Sabin et al., 2007). It may be that such children have higher genetic risk and/or the home environment has greater obesogenic qualities that would impede weight loss compared with their peers with leaner parents. Beyond the parents' weight going into treatment, perhaps one of the most consistent predictors of child weight loss success in the context of family-based treatment is parent weight loss success, such that when the parent is successful, the child is as well (Best et al., 2016; Boutelle et al., 2012; Goldschmidt et al., 2014; Wrotniak, Epstein, Paluch, & Roemmich, 2004). This finding points to the need to encourage behavior change in the family members who surround and influence the child. This point is emphasized by a recent study in which it was shown that the correlation in weight change within child–parent dyads undergoing weight loss treatment could be explained in part by similar dietary changes within the child–parent dyad (Best et al., 2016). This finding suggests that clinicians should help parents and their children create and carry out common strategies to reduce the proportion of energy-dense, nutrient-poor foods in their diets.

When the parent is successful at losing weight, the child typically is as well

Parental feeding practices may also influence children's weight loss success. A restrictive feeding style may actually promote childhood obesity by encouraging a preoccupation with the prohibited food. In the context of family-based obesity treatment, it has been found that reductions in restrictive feeding practices are associated with superior weight loss in children (Cahill Holland et al., 2014; Epstein et al., 2008). These findings are in line with expert committee recommendations that parents avoid overly restrictive feeding practices (Barlow & Expert Committee, 2007).

Restrictive feeding practices may be counterproductive in treating childhood obesity

3.2.3   Psychological and Social Factors

High impulsivity (Best et al., 2012; Nederkoorn, Jansen, Mulkens, & Jansen, 2007) and *greater eating disorder severity* (Wildes et al., 2010), and *poor social functioning* (Goldschmidt et al., 2014) have been shown to be general predictors of poorer weight loss in children. However, weight loss maintenance programs with an explicit focus on eating pathology and related issues (e.g., body image, weigh-related teasing from peers), lead to better outcomes for these children than programs focused solely on self-regulatory and relapse preventions strategies. In addition, weight loss maintenance is improved when parents facilitate positive social supports among peers and within their families and communities, such as planning physically active outings or providing healthy snacks during their child's social activities (Goldschmidt et al., 2014).

3.2.4   Environmental Factors

Just as certain food and built environments may facilitate unhealthy eating and activity patterns, other environments may facilitate healthy behavior change in families participating in treatment for obesity. This is a new area of research that will likely gain greater attention in the near future, but at this time, we are aware of only two studies that address this possibility. In one study (Epstein et al., 2012), children who lived in an area where parkland was abundant, but the presence of supermarkets and convenience stores was low, showed superior long-term weight loss after a family-based treatment. In a more recent study

How the built environment might facilitate or impede weight loss in children is unclear

(Fiechtner et al., 2016), living closer to supermarkets actually predicted greater reductions in relative weight among children. The authors of this second study speculate that the contrasting findings to the previous one might be a result of differing definitions of access to supermarkets. Clearly, more research on how the built environment might impact behavior change within the context of treatment for obesity is warranted, and this future research should pay close attention to how built environment variables are defined.

4

Treatment

4.1 Methods of Treatment

4.1.1 Treatment Guidelines

Organizations and agencies such as the US Preventive Services Task Force (USPSTF) and the AAP have issued guidelines or recommendations for the prevention and treatment of obesity in children (Barlow & Expert Committee, 2007; O'Connor et al., 2017). Additionally, numerous comprehensive reviews and meta-analyses have documented the effectiveness of multicomponent weight loss interventions for children that are of sufficient duration (i.e., greater than 25 hrs of contact), that include a multicomponent focus on diet and physical activity, and that use behavioral change techniques (Janicke et al., 2014; Ho et al., 2012). This chapter provides a brief overview of family-based behavioral weight loss treatments (FBTs) for childhood obesity.

> **The AAP has issued guidelines for the treatment of obesity in children**

4.1.2 Family-Based Treatment

FBTs, developed and expanded upon by Leonard Epstein, Denise Wilfley, and colleagues (Epstein, Paluch, Roemmich, & Beecher, 2007; Wilfley et al., 2007; Wilfley, Saelens, et al., 2017), are consistent with USPSTF and AAP guidelines for treatment of childhood obesity and have demonstrated efficacy in both the short and long term. Modification of energy balance behaviors (i.e., decreasing caloric intake and increasing caloric expenditure) is the cornerstone of many weight loss interventions, including FBT. These goals are achieved through the use of behavioral treatment techniques and the active involvement of a parent or caregiver who often also has overweight or obesity. Appendix 1 provides a brief outline reminder for how to conduct a typical FBT session.

> **FBTs are consistent with national treatment guidelines**

In FBT, the parent is encouraged to modify their own energy balance behaviors, to provide support and encouragement for the child involved in treatment, and to engineer a home environment conducive to a healthy lifestyle for the entire family. It is this focus on change across the entire household that is a hallmark of FBT. Evidence suggests that extended treatment contact focusing on both the continued practice of self-regulatory behavioral skills and the use of family and social networks to support weight loss maintenance behaviors such as improved dietary intake and engagement in increased levels of physical activity is important to the long-term maintenance of weight lost during FBT.

Diet

Dietary targets of FBT include decreasing caloric intake, improving the nutritional quality of foods selected, and shifting food preferences. Decreases in caloric intake of approximately 500 kcal per day from baseline, for a total of 1,000–1,200 kcal per day for children and 1,200–1,400 kcal per day for adults, are achieved by decreasing consumption of high-energy-dense, unhealthy foods, and increasing consumption of nutritious, low-energy-dense foods.

Color-Code Your Food, Make Healthier Choices

Traffic light method provides family-friendly way to categorize foods and make healthier choices

A family-friendly method of categorizing foods according to traffic light colors is used in FBT to help families identify which foods to decrease (Red foods – stop and think; Yellow foods – proceed with caution by watching portion sizes), and which to increase (Green foods – Go!) (Figure 1). Red foods are calorically dense and/or have limited nutritional value (e.g., potato chips, candy, SSBs). Yellow foods are more calorically dense than Green foods but may be more nutritious than Red foods (e.g., whole grain bread), and most vegetables are considered Green foods. The *traffic light* method has helped people change their eating habits, resulting in their choosing more healthful foods (Levy, Riis, Sonnenberg, Barraclough, & Thorndike, 2012; Thorndike, Sonnenberg, Riis, Barraclough, & Levy, 2012; Thorndike, Riis, Sonnenberg, & Levy, 2014).

An important feature of FBT is that caloric reduction is not the only dietary goal; shifting taste preferences is also extremely important. To this end, foods that are modified to be lower in calories (e.g., foods with sugar substitutes such as diet soft drinks, low-fat cookies) are still considered Red foods despite their lower caloric content. The goal of FBT is for families to make a shift to more nutritious foods and not to switch from one "junk" food to a lower calorie version of the same food. In FBT, parental weight loss success predicts child weight loss, and this correlation can be explained, at least in part, by parental maintenance of lower Red food intake over time.

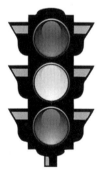

RED
Stop and think
YELLOW
Slow down, caution
GREEN
Go! Best choice

Figure 1
The traffic light method to categorize foods based on their nutritional quality.
(Adapted from Epstein & Squires, 1988)

Another method utilized in FBT for improving the nutritional quality of food and decreasing caloric intake is to encourage families to eat fewer meals away from the home. The average family in the US eats approximately 35% of their meals away from home, and children who have overweight or obesity eat a higher proportion of their meals away from home than children who do not have overweight or obesity. FBT's focus on the reduction of the number of meals eaten away from home has a positive impact not only on participants' weight status but also on the nutritional quality of the foods they eat.

Physical Activity

Physical activity targets in FBT include increasing moderate-to-vigorous physical activity while decreasing time spent in sedentary, non-school or work-related pursuits. The colors of the traffic light again provide a family-friendly way of understanding an activity's intensity or metabolic equivalent (MET). For example, Green activities (Go!) are 5.0 METs or higher; Yellow activities (Slow) are between 3.0 and 4.9 METs, while Red activities (Stop) are less than 3.0 METs. Watching TV, playing video games, talking or texting on the phone, and playing games or "surfing" the Internet on the computer are all Red activities. Any time spent on screen-time activities for a purpose, such as for work or homework, are not counted against Red activity time. Target goals for moderate-to-vigorous physical activity are 60–90 min per day for adults and children. However, FBT also emphasizes the importance of lifestyle physical activities as useful substitutes for sedentary pursuits. For example, walking to the store rather than driving, not only involves more physical activity than driving, but is also more time consuming, thus leaving less time for engaging in computer games or TV watching. Since sedentary activities are often accompanied by eating, decreasing time spent in sedentary pursuits has the added benefit of decreasing caloric intake in addition to increasing caloric output.

FBT targets increases in moderate-to-vigorous physical activity and decreases in sedentary pursuits

Behavior

FBT is a behavioral treatment and the use of behavioral techniques for facilitating change is integral to its successful implementation. Self-monitoring, goal setting, successive approximation and shaping, modeling, and reward systems are the mainstays of good behavioral therapy and are all components of FBT. Self-monitoring has been associated with better weight outcomes in children as well as in adults, and because of this association, it has long been considered one of the most important behavioral change techniques in weight loss interventions. See Appendix 2 for an example of a self-monitoring form that may be adapted and modified for use with children of different developmental levels as well as for use with their parents. Contrary to traditional self-monitoring, which involves recording behaviors after they have occurred, pre-planning is a form of self-monitoring that involves planning or scheduling meals and physical activity a priori. Preplanning may be particularly useful for children with higher impulsivity because it allows families to determine ahead of time how they plan to improve their dietary quality and to increase physical activity. Part of the process of preplanning is developing methods for dealing with potential challenges or barriers to achieving the desired healthy lifestyle behaviors. Appendix 3 offers an example of self-monitoring forms useful in helping families preplan.

FBT is a behavioral intervention

Self-monitoring has been associated with better weight outcomes in children

4.1.3   Social Facilitation Maintenance

Social facilitation maintenance (SFM) is an innovative, socially based behavioral approach to FBT that is developmentally tailored to increase parental support, enhance peer support, improve body image, and teach effective responses to teasing – all strategies for sustaining weight maintenance behaviors. In the first assessment of this intervention informed by a socioenvironmental model delivered in a family-based format, Wilfley and colleagues found that this approach was associated with sustained weight loss compared with a behavioral weight loss intervention and control condition (Wilfley et al., 2007). The socioenvironmental model used increases the duration and extends the scope of standard behavioral weight loss treatment by focusing on practicing skills and infusing support across contexts. This framework encourages behavior change via continued practice of newly learned behaviors throughout a variety of settings. In standard behavioral weight loss intervention, individuals are encouraged to increase their daily physical activity (e.g., go for a run); the socioenvironmental approach builds on this by promoting the engagement of parents and their children in identifying barriers and opportunities in their home and broader community for engagement in healthy lifestyle behaviors. For example, parents are encouraged to offer healthy snacks at their family's various social activities, to facilitate their child in joining sports teams at school, doing physical activity fitness classes with friends, and training for community-based runs (e.g., 5-km events) with their family. Parents are also encouraged to model harnessing social support by engaging in these behaviors/activities themselves. Beyond relying on individual willpower and self-regulatory skills, utilizing the socioenvironmental framework promotes an increased awareness of environmental cues and advocacy for making sustainable healthful changes. For instance, parents will be able to recognize that their usual drive home passes many fast food restaurants that prompt their children to ask for snacks and will be able to select an alternate route to avoid the prompts altogether. Recent evidence supports this approach as a strategy to achieve sustainable weight loss in children and adults. Appendix 4 provides an example of a useful tool for assessing multiple socioenvironmental contexts to facilitate treatment planning and goal setting with families.

4.1.4   Pharmacotherapy

Weight loss medication for the treatment of pediatric obesity may be an acceptable option for select patients when used in combination with lifestyle modifications (Spear et al., 2007), and the urgency to treat severe obesity early may offset the risks associated with pharmacotherapy. However, guidelines for the treatment of pediatric obesity recommend the use of drug therapy only as a final option after comprehensive lifestyle interventions under the supervision of a physician have failed (Expert Panel on Integrated Guidelines for Cardiovascular Health and Risk Reduction in Children and Adolescents & National Heart, Lung, and Blood Institute, 2011). The data assessing the efficacy and safety of pharmacotherapy in adolescents are insufficient, and more high-quality studies are needed. The majority of research has been conducted on three drugs: sibutramine, orlistat, and metformin. Sibutramine was removed from the market in 2012 because of an increased risk of cardiovascular events. Currently, orlistat is the only drug approved in the US for the treatment of obesity in youths aged ≥ 12 years.

Orlistat was approved in 2003 for use in adolescents aged 12–18 years with a BMI > 2 above the reference value at the 95th percentile for age and sex (US Food and Drug Administration, 2003). The medication is sold under the brand names Xenical (prescription) and Alli (over-the-counter), the difference between the two being the dose (120 mg and 60 mg, respectively). Orlistat has a modest impact on weight loss, with approximately 20–25% of patients achieving a 5% weight loss after receiving treatment for 1 year. However, a recent meta-analysis concluded that treatment with orlistat in combination with behavioral intervention was as effective as behavioral intervention alone (Peirson et al., 2015).

Orlistat is the only medication approved to treat childhood obesity

Orlistat functions as a lipase inhibitor, suppressing the action of pancreatic lipase, the enzyme responsible for the breakdown of triglycerides, the form of fat in the diet. Without functional lipase, dietary fats cannot be absorbed in the body and remain in the intestine. As much as one third of the dietary fat can be blocked from absorption (Genentech, 2010). These undigested fats cause gastrointestinal discomfort and are responsible for the most commonly reported side effects including steatorrhea (loose, oily stool), flatulence, abdominal cramping, bloating, and fecal urgency. Symptoms increase as dietary fat intake increases, which acts to negatively reinforce the consumption of high-fat foods. Patients are advised to consume a low-fat diet during therapy as part of their lifestyle modifications but also to reduce uncomfortable side effects. Due to the nature of the side effects, discontinuation rates in adolescents are high (White et al., 2015).

Orlistat is a lipase inhibitor preventing the digestion and absorption of dietary fats

Orlistat has been generally considered safe, with a strong safety record in published clinical trials (Iughetti, China, Berri, & Predieri, 2011). The drug is poorly absorbed and minimally metabolized by the body (Genentech, 2010). However, due to the malabsorptive mechanism of action, orlistat may influence the absorption of the fat-soluble vitamins. Patients taking orlistat are advised to supplement with vitamins A, D, E, and K, consuming the vitamins 2 hrs before orlistat administration. In 2010, the US Food and Drug Administration issued a drug safety communication warning of the risk of severe liver injury, which was reported in rare cases (US Food and Drug Administration, 2010). Signs of severe liver injury include itching, yellow eyes or skin, fever, weakness, vomiting, fatigue, dark urine, light-colored stools, or loss of appetite; if experienced, these symptoms warrant immediate contact with a health care provider. Orlistat is contraindicated for chronic malabsorption syndromes, cholestasis, and pregnancy, and orlistat may interact and weaken the effectiveness of cyclosporin, levothyroxine, warfarin, amiodarone, and antiepileptic drugs. Additional evidence of kidney stones and pancreatitis has also been reported in the literature and are included as potential risks on the warning label. If patients do not respond to treatment with a ≥ 5% weight loss, discontinuation of drug therapy is recommended to decrease risk exposure.

Metformin, a medication used for the management of type 2 diabetes, has been prescribed for off-label use to treat pre-diabetes and insulin resistance with beneficial effects on weight (McDonagh, Selph, Ozpinar, & Foley, 2014).

The prescription of metformin for obesity in the absence of these conditions is discouraged. Metformin reduces gluconeogenesis, or the production of glucose in the liver. Metformin appears to be well tolerated with few adverse events, the most commonly reported complaint being gastrointestinal events. Weight loss with metformin is modest; however, because of its mechanism of action, metformin improves insulin resistance and hyperglycemia, possibly preventing the progression to type 2 diabetes (Bouza, Lopez-Cuadrado, Gutierrez-Torres, & Amate, 2012). In a meta-analysis of 14 trials, McDonagh et al. (2014) reported that metformin in combination with lifestyle interventions modestly reduced BMI and weight, achieving only a 3.6% weight loss, which is less than the clinically significant 5–10%. Thus, metformin may be more effective for patients showing signs of pre–diabetes and insulin resistance and should not be prescribed for obesity without signs of these conditions.

Pharmacotherapy should be used in conjunction with lifestyle change interventions

In summary, the use of drugs for the treatment of pediatric obesity should be limited to those patients who have not responded to other forms of treatment, and as an adjunct to multidisciplinary lifestyle treatment. Orlistat is the only medication approved for the treatment of obesity in adolescents at the time of this publication. However, orlistat has established only a modest effect on weight loss in the treatment of pediatric obesity (O'Connor et al., 2017). Caution should be taken when prescribing drugs to children or adolescents as the long-term consequences of these drug therapies have not yet been evaluated.

4.1.5   Surgical Treatments

Surgical treatment of childhood obesity is controversial

Another treatment option for persistent pediatric obesity caused by dietary and physical activity factors is *bariatric surgery*. Despite the lack of evidence from well-designed studies documenting safety and long-term outcomes, the incidence of bariatric surgeries performed in pediatric populations has steadily increased (Zwintscher, Azarow, Horton, Newton, & Martin, 2013). However, the use of surgical procedures in children is controversial. A variety of adverse events, including severe complications such as pulmonary embolism, severe malnutrition, immediate postoperative bleeding, gastrointestinal obstruction, and postoperative death, have been reported (Treadwell, Sun, & Schoelles, 2008). Because of these risks, experts recommend that the use of bariatric surgery in pediatric patients be limited to adolescents with severe obesity and associated comorbidities (August et al., 2008). A list of specific recommendations for acceptable candidates is seen in Box 5.

Box 5
Bariatric Surgery Recommendations for Adolescents

Conditions for candidacy

Having attained Tanner 4 or 5 pubertal development and final or near-final adult height

- BMI > 50
- BMI > 40 with severe comorbidities
- Severe obesity and comorbidities persist despite a formal lifestyle modification program, with or without trial of pharmacotherapy

- Psychological evaluation confirms the stability and competence of the family unit
- Access to experienced surgeons and a multidisciplinary team capable of long-term follow-up of the metabolic and psychosocial needs of patient and family
- Patient demonstrates ability to adhere to principles of healthy dietary and activity habits

Contraindicated for

- Preadolescent children
- Pregnant or breastfeeding adolescents, and for those planning to become pregnant within 2 years of surgery
- Patients with unresolved eating disorders
- Patients with untreated psychiatric disorders
- Patients with Prader-Willi syndrome Any patient unable to follow healthy dietary and activity habits

There are four general types of bariatric procedures that are currently performed (see Figure 2). *Biliopancreatic diversion with duodenal switch* is considered a malabsorptive procedure, as it bypasses a large portion of the small intestine, which decreases the absorption of nutrients across the intestinal wall. This procedure has a high morbidity and mortality rate and is not recommended for youths (August et al., 2008). A laparoscopic *adjustable gastric band*, the *Roux-en-Y gastric bypass* procedure, and *vertical sleeve gastrectomy* are restrictive procedures that reduce the size of the stomach. The Roux-en-Y gastric bypass also has a malabsorptive effect due to the bypassing of the first part of the intestine, the duodenum. Of these three, an adjustable gastric band is considered the safest and most appropriate for use in children because of the reversible nature of the method and lower risk of severe complications (O'Neil et al., 2014).

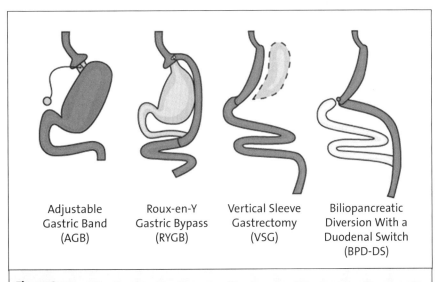

Adjustable Gastric Band (AGB)	Roux-en-Y Gastric Bypass (RYGB)	Vertical Sleeve Gastrectomy (VSG)	Biliopancreatic Diversion With a Duodenal Switch (BPD-DS)

Figure 2
Surgical options for obesity. Image from Walter Pories, MD, FACS. (Source: Wolfe, Kvach, & Eckel, 2016. Reprinted by permission)

Surgical manipulation of the digestive tract impairs the digestion and absorption of nutrients, which is of significant concern in pediatric populations because they are experiencing critical periods of growth and development. The reduced capacity of the stomach and subsequent dramatic reduction of fluid and food intake puts patients at risk for dehydration and protein-energy malnutrition. Common vitamin and mineral deficiencies include those of thiamine (B1), pyridoxine (B6), folic acid (B9), cyanocobalamin (B12), vitamin A, calcium, vitamin D, vitamin C, vitamin E, zinc, magnesium, iron, and copper. To maintain adequate nutritional status, patients must adhere to a strict dietary protocol in the immediate postsurgical period, paying special attention to the type of food, the volume of food and fluid, and the frequency of eating occasions. Supplementation and long-term monitoring of critical nutrients is recommended (Fullmer et al., 2012).

The impact of surgical treatments on psychological well-being is also of critical importance and has not been thoroughly evaluated. Current evidence suggests that adolescents who receive bariatric surgery experience improvements in quality of life and depressive symptoms (Herget, Rudolph, Hilbert, & Bluher, 2014; Jarvholm et al., 2012). Yet, small subpopulations may experience a decline in psychological functioning postsurgery; the reasons for this differential response to treatment have not been identified (Jarvholm et al., 2012). Some studies suggest the improvements in psychosocial functioning and weight wane over time, indicating the positive effects may be of a transient nature (Zeller, Reiter-Purtill, Ratcliff, Inge, & Noll, 2011). Psychological status prior to surgery must also be assessed, as it may complicate adherence to treatment regimens and affect postsurgical outcomes (Herget et al., 2014). Adolescent patients seeking treatment for obesity frequently present with psychopathologies such as depression, anxiety, and disordered eating. Research to date is limited, and clearly defined psychological predictors of treatment success have not been identified (Herget et al., 2014).

The decision to undergo bariatric surgery as a treatment option for pediatric obesity should be thoroughly deliberated. Patients should receive a full physical and psychological health evaluation and be treated in a regional pediatric academic center by a multidisciplinary team able to provide long-term monitoring of medical and psychological status with special attention to nutrient deficiencies (August et al., 2008). Families should be well informed of the risks and complications and the commitment required to implement the necessary lifestyle modifications after the procedure. An important component of treatment success is the full participation of the patient, the family, and the medical team (Shrewsbury, Steinbeck, Torvaldsen, & Baur, 2011).

Bariatric surgery is a life-changing procedure that may be a viable treatment option for a specific segment of adolescents with obesity. Families should be well informed of the full range of risks and benefits before making the decision. While the results from short- to moderate-term studies indicate that bariatric surgery performed in youth may result in improvements in physical and psychological well-being, data from long-term studies are necessary to ensure that the impact on physical and mental health over a lifetime remains positive. Ongoing studies, including the Teen Longitudinal Assessment of bariatric surgery study, a prospective investigation of the safety and efficacy of bariatric surgery in adolescents, have been designed to address these gaps (Michalsky et al., 2014).

4.2   Prevention

Childhood obesity represents an important point of intervention for preventing adult obesity and associated complications, and there has been increased interest in the development of school- and community-based prevention programs. However, universal prevention programs have shown limited efficacy, likely due to the limited focus on individual- or family-level behaviors. Thus, a selective approach may be more efficient. Unlike universal prevention, which involves populations as a whole, indicated prevention involves youths who already have overweight or obesity and thus more likely to track their excess weight into adulthood. Targeting these children is recommended for many reasons. Children are often more successful in weight control programs than adults, perhaps because their dietary and physical activity habits are less ingrained and more amenable to change. Given associations between duration of obesity and adverse medical consequences, children may be less likely than adults to present with comorbidities that could complicate treatment. Finally, interventionists can take advantage of children's concomitant height growth, such that relatively modest weight changes are needed to produce significant reductions in markers of overweight status. For these reasons, targeted intervention approaches may be most efficacious for preventing adult obesity.

4.3   Mechanisms of Action

Although FBTs for childhood obesity result in significant weight loss for both children and participating parents in the short and long term, the mechanisms by which these results are achieved are still unknown. Most programs are multicomponent, focusing on dietary, physical activity, behavioral, and psychosocial changes; however, the precise components or targets that are integral to weight loss have yet to be determined (O'Connor et al., 2017). Research into the mediators and moderators of change can give us some idea of the mechanisms of action (Kazdin, 2007), but to date most of the research into mechanisms of action for weight loss interventions comes from studies with adults. Nonetheless, this research, along with preliminary data from studies with children, can provide some clues as to which program components contribute to successful weight loss in family-based interventions.

Most research on mechanisms of action for weight loss comes from the adult literature

In their systematic review of mediators, Teixeira and colleagues (2015) found that autonomous motivation, self-efficacy, lower perceived barriers, self-regulation skills (e.g., self-monitoring), flexible eating restraint, and positive body image mediated weight control for adults over the medium and long term. The few studies of predictors or mediators of weight loss in FBTs provide results consistent with the findings of the systematic review of Teixeira et al. (2015). For example, in their study of a FBT program targeting children aged

7–11 years, Cahill Holland et al. (2014) found that decreasing parental feeding restrictiveness was associated with reductions in child relative weight and that this mediated decreases in child energy intake. Those parents who were able to help their children decrease their energy intake in a nonrestrictive manner helped reduce their children's degree of overweight; this finding is consistent with the conclusion of Teixeira et al. (2015) that flexible eating restraint is a promising mechanism contributing to successful weight loss in adults.

In addition, self-regulatory skills predict, or mediate, pediatric weight control outcomes in studies of FBT programs. Theim and colleagues (2013) reported that for children 7–12 years of age, self-regulatory and goal-setting skills predicted child weight loss outcomes at 2-year follow-up. In addition, data from a large, multisite trial of an extended FBT program for children aged 7–11 years conducted by Wilfley, Saelens, and colleagues (2017), found that self-regulatory skills such as continued self-monitoring and goal setting according to parental self-report mediated child weight control.

Parental engineering of the home and peer support are promising components of successful programs

The Wilfley, Saelens, et al. (2017) study also found that healthy home environments – in which parents use nonrestrictive feeding practices among other positive parenting techniques – and child healthy behaviors with peers mediated weight loss outcomes. An important component of FBT programs that may allow parents to use nonrestrictive feeding practices is the engineering of the home environment to increase the availability of nutritious foods, along with decreasing the availability of nonnutritious foods. In this way, lower-energy-dense, nutritious food choices become the easier choices for all family members, not just the target child. Given the deleterious effects of body shape and weight stigma, this study also suggests that training in how to deal effectively with teasing and in methods to garner peer support for healthy lifestyle behaviors are mechanisms by which to achieve successful long-term weight control for children.

4.4   Efficacy and Prognosis

The greater the number of contact hours in an intervention, the better the treatment response

The efficacy of family-based, multicomponent behavioral interventions for the treatment of childhood obesity has been well documented. Most recently, a systematic review of the evidence, conducted for the US USPSTF (O'Connor et al., 2017), concluded that lifestyle-based weight loss interventions with 26 or more hours of intervention contact were effective for reducing excess weight in children and adolescents. However, average effect sizes were modest and highly variable with a reduction of relative BMI z score of 0.20 or more found to be the most typical outcome. The only intervention characteristic correlated to effect size was hours of contact; interventions with the greater number of contact hours also had larger effect sizes.

While most studies of FBT programs are limited to 1- or 2-year follow-ups, Epstein and colleagues (Epstein, Valoski, Wing, & McCurley, 1990) conducted a 10-year follow-up of children who had participated in their comprehensive, FBT programs. They found significant differences in weight between treated children and controls at 5- and 10-year follow-up, indicating that the positive outcomes achieved by treating children with obesity can extend into young adulthood. Despite these promising findings, over half of children treated for obesity either do not respond well to initial treatment or fail to maintain improvement in weight status over time (Epstein et al., 1990; O'Connor et al., 2017) suggesting that there are still challenges to effectively treating children who have already converted to having an obese weight status.

4.5   Variations and Combinations of Methods

Most studies of FBT have taken place in specialty academic research centers, but clinical researchers have begun to test the effectiveness of these interventions in alternative settings (e.g., primary care practices) and with alternative delivery methods (e.g., telephonic contacts), and/or with different treatment modalities (e.g., group sessions) are being explored and have shown preliminary promise particularly when very young children at risk for overweight are the target population (Quattrin et al., 2014).

Weight loss interventions for children and their families may be conducted in groups (i.e., multifamily groups and/or child-only and parent-only groups) in an effort to extend the reach and maximize the treatment providers' time investment, but weight loss results are better when families are treated individually and/or with a combination of individual family and group sessions (Hayes, Altman, Coppock, Wilfley, & Goldschmidt, 2015). Greater weight losses when families are treated individually may be the result of better implementation of the behavioral change components of FBT when the focus is on an individual family's unique barriers and strengths rather than trying to address global challenges or issues related to successful weight loss in the group setting (Hayes et al., 2015).

> Treating individual families leads to better treatment outcomes compared with group-only treatments

A potential advantage of these alternative treatment approaches is the ability to reach more youths in need of weight loss services, often in a more cost-efficient manner. Future research is needed to determine the potential clinical advantages of smaller effect sizes across more individuals versus larger effect sizes but with a smaller reach (Epstein et al., 2007; Ma & Frick, 2011). Additionally, methods for augmenting treatment outcomes when delivering pediatric weight control interventions via alternative modalities or in fast-paced clinical settings are being explored and have shown preliminary promise particularly when very young children at risk for overweight are the target population (Quattrin et al., 2014).

4.6   Problems Carrying Out Treatments (Implementation)

Problems participating in and implementing these effective weight control treatments occur across individual, family, societal, and health care policy levels. Making lifestyle changes is difficult in our current obesogenic environment especially given socioeconomic disparities in the availability of, and access to, resources and quality health care. Furthermore, parents may not fully appreciate the serious health consequences of untreated obesity, making it difficult to engage families and youths in much-needed treatment. Even when obesity causes significant distress, internalized obesity stigma and shame may make it challenging for families to request and/or accept treatment (Smith, Straker, McManus, & Fenner, 2014).

Systemic and policy barriers to a wider spread of implementation of these effective weight loss treatments for youths, include lack of a trained workforce to deliver the interventions with high treatment integrity and lack of reimbursement for these types of behavioral health interventions in the current health care marketplace (Wilfley, Staiano, et al., 2017). To date, most training to deliver FBT programs to children has occurred within the context of larger, clinical trials rather than as part of an integrated course of instruction in university or professional schools for health and mental health care providers. In these studies, carefully selected interventionists are trained using a combination of didactic and experiential techniques to deliver the desired intervention with competence and to a high degree of fidelity to the intervention as designed. When such training methods are utilized, outcomes are generally robust and replicable across multiple sites or clinics (e.g., Wilfley, Saelens, et al., 2017). Unfortunately, one reason training in family-based obesity interventions is not prioritized is due to low reimbursement for behavioral health interventions in our current health care system, creating a lack of marketplace incentives for training in this effective treatment method.

With adults, large community programs such as those of the YMCA have joined forces with the CDC to identify, train, and support interventionists to deliver the Diabetes Prevention Program's lifestyle program to adult members of the YMCA. Such partnerships may prove fruitful in ensuring future more widely spread availability of a trained workforce to effectively deliver FBT programs to youths in need (Wilfley, Staiano, et al., 2017). Also, professional organizations are beginning to offer resources and additional training in integrated behavioral health care interventions to their membership, which may lead to greater availability of providers trained to address the serious public health burden of obesity across a variety of treatment settings and age groups (Zeiss, 2016).

4.7   Multicultural Issues

Ethnic minority children and adolescents are disproportionately affected by obesity

As mentioned in Section 1.3, ethnic minority children and adolescents are disproportionately affected by obesity. According to the most recent data, Hispanic children aged 2–19 years have the highest obesity rates (21.9%), followed by non-Hispanic Blacks (19.5%), non-Hispanic Whites (14.7%), and non-Hispanic Asians (8.6%) (Ogden et al., 2016). Reasons for the observed differences in obesity prevalence by ethnicity are likely to be multifaceted, resulting from the combined influence of genetics, culture, and socioeconomic status. However, the foremost contributory factor to high rates of obesity in ethnic minority populations may be socioeconomic status. In a study of over 100,000 students in Grades 1–10, Rogers et al. (2015) reported that the relationship between overweight or obese status and race and ethnicity disappeared after accounting for socioeconomic status. In concordance with this finding, Ogden et al. (2016) found that children residing in homes with a head of household with a high school degree or less had higher rates of obesity compared with those in homes headed by individuals with greater than a high school degree (21% vs. 14%, respectively). Thus many of the barriers to successful treatment in ethnic populations are likely a consequence of socioeconomic status.

Despite differences in obesity prevalence, there is little evidence (as reported above in Section 3.2.1) that treatment outcomes vary by ethnicity. However, multiple barriers to the treatment of low-income, multicultural populations have been reported. For example, treatment attrition is typically higher for ethnic minorities, lower-income, and single-parent families (Kelleher et al., 2017; Williams et al., 2010). Perceived financial costs, lack of transportation and/or child care, and limited time and energy owing to long work hours and multiple jobs are frequently reported as reasons for dropping out of treatment prematurely (Cason-Wilkerson, Goldberg, Albright, Allison, & Haemer, 2015). Additionally, lower-income families may fail to comply with treatment recommendations, due to limited resources for, or access to, healthy foods, lack of health-related knowledge, or an absence of safe spaces for outdoor physical activities. Cultural differences in the perception of overweight are also factors in seeking and maintaining care. Some parents fail to see that their child has a problem with their weight, and may feel that excess weight is a sign of good health (Caprio et al., 2008; Kelleher et al., 2017). These factors are important considerations for clinicians when treating minority populations.

5

Case Vignette

This case vignette is adapted with permission from "Little Big Kids: We Have the Tools to Combat Childhood Obesity, But Lack the Will of Implementation," by E. E. Fitzsimmons-Craft & D. E. Wilfley, 2015, May 8. Available online at *The Common Reader,* http://commonreader.wustl.edu/c/little-big-kids

By the age of 12 years, Amber, who was an only child and lived with her mother, Veronica, had already struggled with the psychosocial and behavioral effects of obesity for several years. Amber was teased remorselessly by peers at school. She felt down about herself and lonely much of the time, and she had a very negative body image. She avoided changing clothes in the school locker room or exposing her body in public. Despite participating on the basketball team at her school, Amber felt completely isolated. She would come home right after school or basketball practice and watch TV and eat sweets and other easily accessible junk food. Because of this pattern, Amber was often up late, scrambling to finish homework.

Nearly everyone in Amber's family struggled with obesity, including her mother. Amber's mother was a single parent who juggled two jobs while raising her daughter. She felt overburdened, isolated, and alone. Pressured by her work schedule, Veronica, frequently sleep deprived, found herself picking up fast food for dinner and stocking the home with easy-to-grab snack foods. Veronica lacked the time, energy, or any sense of incentive, to plan and prepare home-cooked meals. When she did have a spare moment, she found herself watching TV and eating foods such as chips and cookies to unwind from her hectic day. Given her own habits and feelings of guilt for not having enough time for Amber, it was hard for Veronica to say no to Amber when she requested fast food, or to set limits with her about bedtime.

Despite the fact that Amber had struggled with the effects of excessive weight for many years, Veronica was first informed that her daughter's weight was in the obese category and that she was at high risk for the development of type 2 diabetes, at Amber's 12-year-old check-up. Veronica was shocked to learn that the problem was so critical and was upset that her daughter's pediatrician had not warned her sooner. Veronica was given some educational materials on childhood obesity, nutrition, and physical activity; however, she did not have a plan or strategy to help her daughter achieve a healthier weight. She felt despair and anger that she had somehow failed as a parent. Fortunately, Amber's pediatrician also referred Amber and her mother to a university-based clinical trial testing weight control interventions for children and their families.

For Amber and Veronica, the family-based behavioral treatment they participated in ultimately helped them to reduce unhealthy habits associated with weight gain and to increase sustainable, health-promoting skills and behaviors. First, their family interventionist worked with them to understand the problem, what contributes to excessive weight gain, and why in our obesogenic environment it is difficult to maintain a healthy weight. They identified the times when Amber was most likely to overeat and other factors that maintained the family's unhealthy habits, as well as the family's strengths and resources. By taking a careful history and reviewing Amber's health records, their interventionist learned that although Amber had always been a heavy child, her weight had likely moved into the obese range about 3 years ago – a time that coincided with her parents' divorce. In addition to overeating after school when she was home alone, other factors that were identified as contributing to the problem included lack of time, social isolation, keeping junk food in the home, lack of scheduled eating times, and lack of easy access to a grocery store.

After gaining a thorough understanding of contributors to the problem, the interventionist collaborated with the family to create intervention goals and to design gradual ways to make durable changes in order to achieve these goals. For example, one of the first things the family worked on was implementing more planned, regular eating – three meals and one to two snacks each day. Given Veronica's extremely busy work schedule and the fact that there was not a grocery store nearby, this was not easy, but the family got creative to make it work. They learned which healthy, affordable staples would last and could be cooked quickly, like oatmeal, eggs, beans, and frozen fruits and vegetables. When they were able to get to the grocery store once or twice a month or when there were sales, they stocked up on these items. They worked out a way to eat breakfast together most days of the week and learned to pack affordable, healthful lunches and snacks for school and work.

Dinner and the time after Amber got home from school remained challenging, though, as Veronica sometimes had to work late. Veronica was able arrange for Amber to go to her sister's house several days per week, which also afforded Amber the opportunity to spend some time with her two younger cousins. However, Veronica's sister did not always serve the most nutritious foods – Veronica recruited her sister as an advocate for their children's health by helping her understand the importance of disease prevention through healthy lifestyle changes. In this way, Veronica's sister was helping not only Amber but also her own family. On days when Amber was home alone, Veronica made sure there were quick, healthful dinners available, and she minimized the amount of junk food kept in the home. Veronica also learned the importance of having plenty of alternative activities for Amber at home too, like books and puzzles, so that Amber would be less likely to eat to deal with boredom.

It took practice for Veronica to make healthy eating a priority for herself – it was not always easy to resist fast food, and she sometimes slipped, but she was ultimately able to change this habit by reminding herself that getting healthy meant that she would be there for her daughter in the long term. The family learned that while they did not need to cut out favorite foods like chips and cookies completely, it was important to treat these as "sometimes" rather than "always" foods. As they were working on improving their eating, Amber and Veronica also worked to implement other lifestyle changes – for example, doing something really active together on the weekend, like swimming or playing soccer, and walking together in the evening whenever possible. Veronica learned that a few of her neighbors were also trying to lose weight and invited these neighbors and their children to join them in their evening or weekend physical activities. By reaching out in this way, Amber and Veronica were able to build a peer network supportive of healthy lifestyle activities.

With practice, both Amber and Veronica were also able to get their sleep on track. Then, to join her mother or neighborhood friends in their evening activities, Amber learned to do her homework right after school. Also, once Veronica prioritized getting up in the morning to have breakfast with Amber, and after she became more active with more outside-of-work social interactions, Veronica no longer felt the need to stay up late watching TV each evening.

Gradually, by implementing these changes, Amber's weight became more appropriate for her height, and her risk for type 2 diabetes decreased. She also saw that it became easier for her to play basketball and be active; these changes increased her body esteem, making it easier for her to play with her peers at school and in the neighborhood and to improve her social relationships. Amber and Veronica even became advocates for healthy living at Amber's school – for example, by petitioning for the availability of more healthy foods in the cafeteria so that all of the children and staff at the school could enjoy a healthier lifestyle.

6

Further Reading

Bradley, D. W., Dietz, W. H., & the Provider Training and Education Workgroup. (June, 2017). *Provider competencies for the prevention and management of obesity.* Washington, DC: Bipartisan Policy Center. Retrieved from https://bipartisanpolicy.org/library/provider-competencies-for-the-prevention-and-management-of-obesity
This collaborative effort between the Bipartisan Policy Center and more than 20 leading health organizations representing a dozen health professions (including the American Psychological Association) outlines core competencies regarding obesity prevention and management for adults. Although not meant to be a comprehensive curriculum, this publication seeks to begin to close the training gap that exists for the many health professionals working with obesity, the majority of whom feel inadequately trained to provide nutritional and physical activity counseling to their patients.

Centers for Disease Control and Prevention. (2017). *Growth charts for diagnosing obesity in children.* Retrieved from https://www.cdc.gov/growthcharts/clinical_charts.htm

Daniels, S.R., & Hassink, S. (2015). The role of the pediatrician in primary prevention of obesity. *Pediatrics, 136*(1), e275–e292. https://doi.org/10.1542/peds.2015-1558
This commentary provides a rationale for integrating primary prevention of obesity into pediatric practices. Useful descriptions of the prevention goals and strategies for use within busy pediatric practices are included. Areas in need of further research are also discussed.

Epstein, L., & Squires, S. (1988). *The stoplight diet for children: An eight-week program for parents and children.* New York, NY: Little, Brown and Company.
This classic book describes the foundational family-based behavioral weight loss program pioneered by Dr. Epstein and colleagues. Although the intervention has evolved over the years in response to new research in the social, cognitive, and behavioral sciences, this book introduces the basics of taking a family-based approach to weight loss for children.

Quattrin, T., & Wilfley, D. E. (2017). The promise and opportunities for screening and treating childhood obesity. *JAMA Pediatrics, 171*(8), 733–735. https://doi.org/10.1001/jamapediatrics.2017.1604
This commentary summarizes the guidelines for screening and treating childhood obesity put forth by the US Preventive Services Task Force. The authors also review some of the key issues related to implementation of these guidelines, including the advantages of incorporating behavioral specialists into patient-centered medical homes for addressing the growing problem of childhood obesity.

Treatment Options for Type 2 Diabetes in Adolescents and Youth (TODAY) Study. (n.d.) Retrieved from https://today.bsc.gwu.edu/web/today/home?p_p_id=58&p_p_lifecycle=0&_58_redirect=%2F
This website provides access to educational materials and handouts (English and Spanish versions) designed specifically to promote healthy lifestyles and weight loss for children and youth with recent onset type 2 diabetes, and their families. Although participants in the lifestyle intervention did not achieve better glycemic control than those in the medication-only arms, they did achieve superior weight loss outcomes during

the first 6 months of the study, which was the time in the study with the most intensive treatment contact (i.e., weekly, in-person family sessions).

US Preventive Services Task Force et al. (2017). Screening for obesity in children and adolescents: US Preventive Services Task Force recommendation statement. *JAMA, 317*(23), 2417–2426. https://doi.org/10.1001/jama.2017.6803
This article reports on the findings of the USPSTF's most recent review of the pediatric obesity treatment literature and outlines recommendations for length and intensity of treatment associated with best clinical outcomes.

World Health Organization. (n.d.). *Child growth standards ages 0–19.* Retrieved from http://www.who.int/childgrowth/en/
These resources link to the growth charts referred to in Sections 1.2 "Definition" and 1.7 "Diagnostic Procedures and Documentation," as well as in Table 1.

7

References

Allison, D. B., Downey, M., Atkinson, R. L., Billington, C. J., Bray, G. A., Eckel, R. H., … Tremblay, A. (2008). Obesity as a disease: A white paper on evidence and arguments commissioned by the Council of the Obesity Society. *Obesity, 16*(6), 1161–1177. https://doi.org/10.1038/oby.2008.231

Allison, D. B., Kaprio, J., Korkeila, M., Koskenvuo, M., Neale, M. C., & Hayakawa, K. (1996). The heritability of body mass index among an international sample of monozygotic twins reared apart. *International Journal of Obesity, 20*, 501–506.

Altman, M., Cahill Holland, J., Lundeen, D., Kolko, R. P., Stein, R. I., Saelens, B. E., … Wilfley, D. E. (2015). Reduction in food away from home is associated with improved child relative weight and body composition outcomes and this relation is mediated by changes in diet quality. *Journal of the Academy of Nutrition and Dietetics, 115*(9), 1400–1407. http://doi.org/10.1016/j.jand.2015.03.009

American Psychiatric Association. (2013). *Diagnostic and statistical manual of mental disorders* (5th ed.). Arlington, VA: American Psychiatric Publishing. http://doi.org/10.1176/appi.books.9780890425596

Appelhans, B. M., Waring, M. E., Schneider, K. L., & Pagoto, S. L. (2014). Food preparation supplies predict children's family meal and home-prepared dinner consumption in low-income households. *Appetite, 76*, 1–8. http://doi.org/10.1016/j.appet.2014.01.008

Archer, E., Shook, R. P., Thomas, D. M., Church, T. S., Katzmarzyk, P. T., Hebert, J. R., … Blair, S. N. (2013). 45-Year trends in women's use of time and household management energy expenditure. *PLoS, 8*(2), e56620. http://doi.org/10.1371/journal.pone.0056620

August, G. P., Caprio, S., Fennoy, I., Freemark, M., Kaufman, F. R., Lustig, R. H., … Montori, V. M. (2008). Prevention and treatment of pediatric obesity: An endocrine society clinical practice guideline based on expert opinion. *The Journal of Clinical Endocrinology and Metabolism, 93*(12), 4576–4599. http://doi.org/10.1210/jc.2007-2458

Ayala, G. X., Rogers, M., Arredondo, E. M., Campbell, N. R., Baquero, B., Duerksen, S. C., & Elder, J. P. (2008). Away-from-home food intake and risk for obesity: Examining the influence of context. *Obesity, 16*(5), 1002–1008. http://doi.org/10.1038/oby.2008.34

Barlow, S. E., & Expert Committee. (2007). Expert committee recommendations regarding the prevention, assessment, and treatment of child and adolescent overweight and obesity: Summary report. *Pediatrics, 120*(Suppl 4), S164–S192. http://doi.org/10.1542/peds.2007-2329C

Berkey, C. S., & Colditz, G. A. (2007). Adiposity in adolescents: Change in actual BMI works better than change in BMI z score for longitudinal studies. *Annals of Epidemiology, 17*(1), 44–50. http://doi.org/10.1016/j.annepidem.2006.07.014

Best, J. R., Goldschmidt, A. B., Mockus-Valenzuela, D. S., Stein, R. I., Epstein, L. H., & Wilfley, D. E. (2016). Shared weight and dietary changes in parent-child dyads following family-based obesity treatment. *Health Psychology, 35*(1), 92–95. http://doi.org/10.1037/hea0000247

Best, J. R., Miller, P. H., & Jones, L. L. (2009). Executive functions after age 5: Changes and correlates. *Developmental Review, 29*, 180–200. http://doi.org/10.1016/j.dr.2009.05.002

Best, J. R., Theim, K. R., Gredysa, D. M., Stein, R. I., Welch, R. R., Saelens, B. E., … Wilfley, D. E. (2012). Behavioral economic predictors of overweight children's weight loss. *Journal of Consulting and Clinical Psychology, 80*(6), 1086–1096. http://doi.org/10.1037/a0029827

Booth, J. N., Tomporowski, P. D., Boyle, J. M., Ness, A. R., Joinson, C., Leary, S. D., & Reilly, J. J. (2013). Associations between executive attention and objectively measured physical activity in adolescence: Findings from ALSPAC, a UK cohort. *Mental Health and Physical Activity, 6*(3), 212–219. http://doi.org/10.1016/j.mhpa.2013.09.002

Borghi, E., de Onis, M., Garza, C., Van den Broeck, J., Frongillo, E. A., Grummer-Strawn, L., … Martines, J. C. (2006). Construction of the World Health Organization child growth standards: Selection of methods for attained growth curves. *Statistics in Medicine, 25*(2), 247–265. http://doi.org/10.1002/sim.2227

Boutelle, K. N., Cafri, G., & Crow, S. J. (2012). Parent predictors of child weight change in family based behavioral obesity treatment. *Obesity, 20*(7), 1539–1543. http://doi.org/10.1038/oby.2012.48

Bouza, C., Lopez-Cuadrado, T., Gutierrez-Torres, L. F., & Amate, J. (2012). Efficacy and safety of metformin for treatment of overweight and obesity in adolescents: An updated systematic review and meta-analysis. *Obesity Facts, 5*(5), 753–765. http://doi.org/10.1159/000345023

Bowman, S. A., Gortmaker, S. L., Ebbeling, C. B., Pereira, M. A., & Ludwig, D. S. (2004). Effects of fast-food consumption on energy intake and diet quality among children in a national household survey. *Pediatrics, 113*(1 Pt 1), 112–118. http://doi.org/10.1542/peds.113.1.112

Cahill Holland, J., Kolko, R. P., Stein, R. I., Welch, R. R., Perri, M. G., Schechtman, K. B., … Wilfley, D. E. (2014). Modifications in parent feeding practices and child diet during family-based behavioral treatment improve child zBMI. *Obesity, 22*(5), E119–E126.

Caprio, S., Daniels, S. R., Drewnowski, A., Kaufman, F. R., Palinkas, L. A., Rosenbloom, A. L., … Kirkman, S. M. (2008). Influence of race, ethnicity, and culture on childhood obesity: Implications for prevention and treatment. *Obesity, 16*(12), 2566–2577. http://doi.org/10.1038/oby.2008.398

Carnell, S., & Wardle, J. (2007). Measuring behavioural susceptibility to obesity: Validation of the child eating behaviour questionnaire. *Appetite, 48*(1), 104–113. http://doi.org/10.1016/j.appet.2006.07.075

Carnell, S., & Wardle, J. (2008). Appetite and adiposity in children: Evidence for a behavioral susceptibility theory of obesity. *The American Journal of Clinical Nutrition, 88*, 22–29.

Cason-Wilkerson, R., Goldberg, S., Albright, K., Allison, M., & Haemer, M. (2015). Factors influencing healthy lifestyle changes: A qualitative look at low-income families engaged in treatment for overweight children. *Childhood Obesity, 11*(2), 170–176. http://doi.org/10.1089/chi.2014.0147

Centers for Disease Control and Prevention. (2003). Physical activity levels among children aged 9–13 years: United States, 2002. *Morbidity and Mortality Weekly Report, 52*(33), 785–788.

Cohen, A. K., Rai, M., Rehkopf, D. H., & Abrams, B. (2013). Educational attainment and obesity: A systematic review. *Obesity Reviews, 14*(12), 989–1005. http://doi.org/10.1111/obr.12062

Cole, T. J., Bellizzi, M. C., Flegal, K. M., & Dietz, W. H. (2000). Establishing a standard definition for child overweight and obesity worldwide: International survey. *BMJ, 320*(7244), 1240–1243.

Coll, A. P., & Loraine Tung, Y. C. (2009). Pro-opiomelanocortin (POMC)-derived peptides and the regulation of energy homeostasis. *Molecular and Cellular Endocrinology, 300* (1–2), 147–151. https://doi.org/10.1016/j.mce.2008.09.007

Cooper, A. R., Goodman, A., Page, A. S., Sherar, L. B., Esliger, D. W., van Sluijs, E. M., … Ekelund, U. (2015). Objectively measured physical activity and sedentary time in youth: The International children's accelerometry database (ICAD). *The International Journal of Behavioral Nutrition and Physical Activity, 12*, 113. http://doi.org/10.1186/s12966-015-0274-5

Council on Sports Medicine and Fitness & Council on School Health. (2006). Active healthy living: Prevention of childhood obesity through increased physical activity. *Pediatrics, 117*(5), 1834–1842. Retrieved from http://pediatrics.aappublications.org/content/pediatrics/117/5/1834.full.pdf http://doi.org/10.1542/peds.2006-0472

Daniel, T. O., Stanton, C. M., & Epstein, L. H. (2013). The future is now: Comparing the effect of episodic future thinking on impulsivity in lean and obese individuals. *Appetite, 71*, 120–125. http://doi.org/10.1016/j.appet.2013.07.010

Datar, A., & Sturm, R. (2006). Childhood overweight and elementary school outcomes. *International Journal of Obesity, 30*, 1449–1460. http://doi.org/10.1038/sj.ijo.0803311

Davidson, T., Kanoski, S., Walls, E., & Jarrard, L. (2005). Memory inhibition and energy regulation. *Physiology & Behavior, 86*(5), 731–746. http://doi.org/10.1016/j.physbeh. 2005.09.004

de Onis, M., Blossner, M., & Borghi, E. (2010). Global prevalence and trends of overweight and obesity among preschool children. *The American Journal of Clinical Nutrition, 92*(5), 1257–1264. http://doi.org/10.3945/ajcn.2010.29786

de Onis, M., Onyango, A. W., Borghi, E., Siyam, A., Nishida, C., & Siekmann, J. (2007). Development of a WHO growth reference for school-aged children and adolescents. *Bulletin of the World Health Organization, 85*(9), 660–667. http://doi.org/10.2471/BLT. 07.043497

de Ruyter, J. C., Olthof, M. R., Seidell, J. C., & Katan, M. B. (2012). A trial of sugar-free or sugar-sweetened beverages and body weight in children. *New England Journal of Medicine, 367*(15), 1397–1406. http://doi.org/10.1056/NEJMoa1203034

Deshmukh-Taskar, P. R., Nicklas, T. A., O'Neil, C. E., Keast, D. R., Radcliffe, J. D., & Cho, S. (2010). The relationship of breakfast skipping and type of breakfast consumption with nutrient intake and weight status in children and adolescents: The National Health and Nutrition Examination Survey 1999–2006. *Journal of the American Dietetic Association, 110*(6), 869–878. http://doi.org/10.1016/j.jada.2010.03.023

Ebbeling, C. B., Feldman, H. A., Chomitz, V. R., Antonelli, T. A., Gormaker, S. L., Osganian, S. K., Ludwig, D. S. (2012). A randomized trial of sugar-sweetened beverages and adolescent body weight. *New England Journal of Medicine, 367*(15), 1407–1416. http:// doi.org/10.1056/NEJMoa1203388

Epstein, L. H., Paluch, R. A., Beecher, M. D., & Roemmich, J. N. (2008). Increasing healthy eating vs. reducing high energy-dense foods to treat pediatric obesity. *Obesity, 16*(2), 318–326. http://doi.org/10.1038/oby.2007.61

Epstein, L. H., Paluch, R. A., & Raynor, H. A. (2001). Sex differences in obese children and siblings in family-based obesity treatment. *Obesity Research, 9*(12), 746–753. http://doi. org/10.1038/oby.2001.103

Epstein, L. H., Paluch, R. A., Roemmich, J. N., & Beecher, M. D. (2007). Family-based obesity treatment, then and now: Twenty-five years of pediatric obesity treatment. *Health Psychology, 26*(4), 381–391. http://doi.org/10.1037/0278-6133.26.4.381

Epstein, L. H., Raja, S., Daniel, T. O., Paluch, R. A., Wilfley, D. E., Saelens, B. E., & Roemmich, J. N. (2012). The built environment moderates effects of family-based childhood obesity treatment over 2 years. *Annals of Behavioral Medicine, 44*(2), 248–258. http://doi.org/10.1007/s12160-012-9383-4

Epstein, L. H., Salvy, S. J., Carr, K. A., Dearing, K. K., & Bickel, W. K. (2010). Food reinforcement, delay discounting and obesity. *Physiology & Behavior, 100*, 438–445. http:// doi.org/10.1016/j.physbeh.2010.04.029

Epstein, L., & Squires, S. (1988). *The stoplight diet for children: An eight-week program for parents and children.* New York, NY: Little, Brown and Company.

Epstein, L. H., Valoski, A., Wing, R. R., & McCurley, J. (1990). Ten-year follow-up of behavioral, family-based treatment for obese children. *Journal of the American Medical Association, 264*, 2519–2523. http://doi.org/10.1001/jama.1990.03450190051027

Expert Panel on Integrated Guidelines for Cardiovascular Health and Risk Reduction in Children and Adolescents & National Heart, Lung, and Blood Institute. (2011). Expert panel on integrated guidelines for cardiovascular health and risk reduction in children and adolescents: Summary report. *Pediatrics, 128*(Suppl 5), S213–S256. http://doi. org/10.1542/peds.2009-2107C

Fiechtner, L., Kleinman, K., Melly, S. J., Sharifi, M., Marshall, R., Block, J., … Taveras, E. M. (2016). Effects of proximity to supermarkets on a randomized trial studying interventions for obesity. *American Journal of Public Health, 106*(3), 557–562. http://doi. org/10.2105/AJPH.2015.302986

Finkelstein, E. A., & Strombotne, K. L. (2010). The economics of obesity. *The American Journal of Clinical Nutrition, 91*(5), 1520S–1524S. http://doi.org/10.3945/ajcn.2010.28701E

Flegal, K. M., Kit, B. K., Orpana, H., & Graubard, B. I. (2013). Association of all-cause mortality with overweight and obesity using standard body mass index categories: A systematic review and meta-analysis. *Journal of the American Medical Association, 309*(1), 71–82. http://doi.org/10.1001/jama.2012.113905

Francis, L. A., & Susman, E. J. (2009). Self-regulation and rapid weight gain in children from age 3 to 12 years. *Archives of Pediatrics & Adolescent Medicine, 163*(4), 297–302. http://doi.org/10.1001/archpediatrics.2008.579

Franks, P. W., Jablonski, K. A., Delahanty, L. M., McAteer, J. B., Kahn, S. E., Knowler, W. C., & Florez, J. C. (2008). Assessing gene-treatment interactions at the FTO and INSIG2 loci on obesity-related traits in the Diabetes Prevention Program. *Diabetologia, 51*(12), 2214–2223. http://doi.org/10.1007/s00125-008-1158-x

Fulkerson, J. A., Farbakhsh, K., Lytle, L., Hearst, M. O., Dengel, D. R., Pasch, K. E., & Kubik, M. Y. (2011). Away-from-home family dinner sources and associations with weight status, body composition, and related biomarkers of chronic disease among adolescents and their parents. *Journal of the American Dietetic Association, 111*(12), 1892–1897. http://doi.org/10.1016/j.jada.2011.09.035

Fullmer, M. A., Abrams, S. H., Hrovat, K., Mooney, L., Scheimann, A. O., Hillman, J. B., & Suskind, D. L. (2012). Nutritional strategy for adolescents undergoing bariatric surgery: report of a working group of the Nutrition Committee of NASPGHAN/NACHRI. *Journal of Pediatric Gastroenterology and Nutrition, 54*(1), 125–135. http://doi.org/10.1097/MPG.0b013e318231db79

Gable, S., Krull, J. L., & Chang, Y. (2012). Boys' and girls' weight status and math performance from kindergarten entry through fifth grade: A mediated analysis. *Child Development, 83*(5), 1822–1839. http://doi.org/10.1111/j.1467-8624.2012.01803.x

Genentech. (2010). *Xenical® (orlistat) capsules* [Package insert]. South San Francisco, CA: Roche. Retrieved from http://www.accessdata.fda.gov/drugsatfda_docs/label/2010/020766s028lbl.pdf

Gioia, G. A., Isquith, P. K., Guy, S. C., & Kenworthy, L. (2000). Behavior Rating Inventory of Executive Function. *Child Neuropsychology, 6*(3), 235–238. http://doi.org/10.1076/chin.6.3.235.3152

Gishti, O., Gaillard, R., Durmus, B., Abrahamse, M., van der Beek, E. M., Holfman, A., … Jaddoe, V. W. (2015). BMI, total and abdominal fat distribution, and cardiovascular risk factors in school-age children. *Pediatric Research, 77*(5), 710–718. http://doi.org/10.1038/pr.2015.29

Goldfield, G. S., Epstein, L., Davidson, M., & Saad, F. (2005). Validation of a questionnaire measure of the relative reinforcing value of food. *Eating Behaviors, 6*, 283–292. http://doi.org/10.1016/j.eatbeh.2004.11.004

Goldschmidt, A. B., Best, J. R., Stein, R. I., Saelens, B. E., Epstein, D. H., & Wilfley, D. E. (2014). Predictors of child weight loss and maintenance among family-based treatment completers. *Journal of Consulting and Clinical Psychology, 82*(6), 1140–1150. http://doi.org/10.1037/a0037169

Goldschmidt, A. B., Wilfley, D. E., Paluch, R. A., Roemmich, J. N., & Epstein, L. H. (2013). Indicated prevention of adult obesity: How much weight change is necessary for normalization of weight status in children? *JAMA Pediatrics, 167*(1), 21–26. http://doi.org/10.1001/jamapediatrics.2013.416

Goodman, E., & Whitaker, R. C. (2002). A prospective study of the role of depression in the development and persistence of adolescent obesity. *Pediatrics, 110*(3), 497–504. http://doi.org/10.1542/peds.110.3.497

Gupta, N., Goel, K., Shah, P., & Misra, A. (2012). Childhood obesity in developing countries: Epidemiology, determinants, and prevention. *Endocrine Reviews, 33*(1), 48–70. 8 http://doi.org/10.1210/er.2010-0028

Guthrie, J. F., Lin, B. H., & Frazao, E. (2002). Role of food prepared away from home in the American diet, 1977-78 versus 1994-96: Changes and consequences. *Journal of*

Nutrition Education and Behavior, 34(3), 140–150. http://doi.org/10.1016/S1499-4046(06)60083-3

Hayes, J. F., Altman, M., Coppock, J. H., Wilfley, D. E., & Goldschmidt, A. B. (2015). Recent updates on the efficacy of group based treatments for pediatric obesity. *Current Cardiovascular Risk Reports, 9*(4), 16. http://doi.org/10.1007/s12170-015-0443-8

Herget, S., Rudolph, A., Hilbert, A., & Bluher, S. (2014). Psychosocial status and mental health in adolescents before and after bariatric surgery: A systematic literature review. *Obesity Facts, 7*(4), 233–245. http://doi.org/10.1159/000365793

Hill, C., Saxton, J., Webber, L., Blundell, J., & Wardle, J. (2009). The relative reinforcing value of food predicts weight gain in a longitudinal study of 7-10-y-old children. *The American Journal of Clinical Nutrition, 90*, 276–281. http://doi.org/10.3945/ajcn.2009.27479

Ho, M., Garnett, S. P., Baur, L., Burrows, T., Stewart, L., Neve, M., & Collins, C. (2012). Effectiveness of lifestyle interventions in child obesity: Systematic review with meta-analysis. *Pediatrics, 130*, e1647–e1671.

Houben, K., & Jansen, A. (2011). Training inhibitory control. A recipe for resisting sweet temptations. *Appetite, 56*(2), 345–349. http://doi.org/10.1016/j.appet.2010.12.017

Huszar, D., Lynch, C. A., Fairchild-Huntress, V., Dunmore, J. H., Fang, Q., Berkemeier, L. R., … Lee, F. (1997). Targeted disruption of the melanocortin-4 receptor results in obesity in mice. *Cell, 88*(1), 131–141. https://doi.org/10.1016/S0092-8674(00)81865-6

Iughetti, L., China, M., Berri, R., & Predieri, B. (2011). Pharmacological treatment of obesity in children and adolescents: Present and future. *Journal of Obesity, 2011*, 928165. http://doi.org/10.1155/2011/928165

Jabs, J., & Devine, C. M. (2006). Time scarcity and food choices: An overview. *Appetite, 47*(2), 196–204. http://doi.org/10.1016/j.appet.2006.02.014

Janicke, D. M., Steele, R. G., Gayes, L. A., Lim, C. S., Clifford, L. M., Schneider, E. M., … Westen, S. (2014). Systematic review and meta-analysis of comprehensive behavioral family lifestyle interventions addressing pediatric obesity. *Journal of Pediatric Psychology, 39*(8), 809–825. http://doi.org/10.1093/jpepsy/jsu023

Jarvholm, K., Olbers, T., Marcus, C., Marild, S., Gronowitz, E., Friberg, P., … Flodmark, C. E. (2012). Short-term psychological outcomes in severely obese adolescents after bariatric surgery. *Obesity (Silver Spring), 20*(2), 318–323. http://doi.org/10.1038/oby.2011.310

Juonala, M., Magnussen, C. G., Berenson, G. S., Venn, A., Burns, T. L., Sabin, M. A., … Raitakari, O. T. (2011). Childhood adiposity, adult adiposity, and cardiovascular risk factors. *New England Journal of Medicine, 365*(20), 1876–1885. http://doi.org/10.1056/NEJMoa1010112

Kazdin, A. E. (2007). Mediators and mechanisms of change in psychotherapy research. *Annual Review of Clinical Psychology, 3*, 1–27. http://doi.org/10.1146/annurev.clinpsy.3.022806.091432

Kelleher, E., Davoren, M. P., Harrington, J. M., Shiely, F., Perry, I. J., & McHugh, S. M. (2017). Barriers and facilitators to initial and continued attendance at community-based lifestyle programmes among families of overweight and obese children: a systematic review. *Obesity Reviews, 18*(2), 183–194. http://doi.org/10.1111/obr.12478

Kit, B. K., Fakhouri, T. H., Park, S., Nielsen, S. J., & Ogden, C. L. (2013). Trends in sugar-sweetened beverage consumption among youth and adults in the United States: 1999–2010. *The American Journal of Clinical Nutrition, 98*(1), 180–188. http://doi.org/10.3945/ajcn.112.057943

Kuczmarski, R. J., Ogden, C. L., Guo, S. S., Grummer-Strawn, L. M., Flegal, K. M., Mei, Z., … Johnson, C. L. (2002). 2000 CDC growth charts for the United States: Methods and development. *Vital and Health Statistics, 11*(246), 1–190.

Leidy, H. J., Hoertel, H. A., Douglas, S. M., Higgins, K. A., & Shafer, R. S. (2015). A high-protein breakfast prevents body fat gain, through reductions in daily intake and hunger, in "Breakfast skipping" adolescents. *Obesity, 23*(9), 1761–1764. http://doi.org/10.1002/oby.21185

Levy, D. E., Riis, J., Sonnenberg, L. M., Barraclough, S. J., & Thorndike, A. N. (2012). Food choices of minority and low-income employees: A cafeteria intervention. *American*

Journal of Preventive Medicine, 43(3), 240–248. http://doi.org/10.1016/j.amepre.2012.05.004

Li, Z., Zhou, Y., Carter-Su, C., Myers, M. G., Jr., & Rui, L. (2007). SH2B1 enhances leptin signaling by both Janus kinase 2 Tyr813 phosphorylation-dependent and –independent mechanisms. *Molecular Endocrinology, 21*(9), 2270–2281. http://doi.org/10.1210/me.2007-0111

Liang, J., Matheson, B. E., Kaye, W. H., & Boutelle, K. N. (2014). Neurocognitive correlates of obesity and obesity-related behaviors in children and adolescents. *International Journal of Obesity, 38*(4), 484–506. http://doi.org/10.1038/ijo.2013.142

Llewellyn, C. H., Trzaskowski, M., Plomin, R., & Wardle, J. (2013). Finding the missing heritability in pediatric obesity: The contribution of genome-wide complex trait analysis. *International Journal of Obesity, 37*(11), 1506–1509. http://doi.org/10.1038/ijo.2013.30

Ludwig, D. S. (2007). Childhood obesity – the shape of things to come. *New England Journal of Medicine, 357*(23), 2325–2327. http://doi.org/10.1056/NEJMp0706538

Lumeng, J. C., Gannon, K., Cabral, H. J., Frank, D. A., & Zuckerman, B. (2003). Association between clinically meaningful behavior problems and overweight in children. *Pediatrics, 112*(5), 1138–1145. http://doi.org/10.1542/peds.112.5.1138

Luppino, F. S., de Wit, L. M., Bouvy, P. F., Stijnen, T., Cuijpers, P., Penninx, B. W., & Zitman, F. G. (2010). Overweight, obesity, and depression: A systematic review and meta-analysis of longitudinal studies. *Archives of General Psychiatry, 67*(3), 220–229. http://doi.org/10.1001/archgenpsychiatry.2010.2

Ma, S., & Frick, K. D. (2011). A simulation of affordability and effectiveness of childhood obesity interventions. *Academic Pediatrics, 11*(4), 342–350. http://doi.org/10.1016/j.acap.2011.04.005

Maffeis, C., Pietrobelli, A., Grezzani, A., Provera, S., & Tato, L. (2001). Waist circumference and cardiovascular risk factors in prepubertal children. *Obesity Research, 9*(3), 179–187. http://doi.org/10.1038/oby.2001.19

Malik, M., & Bakir, A. (2007). Prevalence of overweight and obesity among children in the United Arab Emirates. *Obesity Reviews, 8*(1), 15–20. http://doi.org/10.1111/j.1467-789X.2006.00290.x

Marcus, M. D., & Wildes, J. E. (2012). Obesity in DSM-5. *Psychiatric Annals, 42*, 431–435. http://doi.org/10.3928/00485713-20121105-10

Matthys, C., De Henauw, S., Bellemans, M., De Maeyer, M., & De Backer, G. (2007). Breakfast habits affect overall nutrient profiles in adolescents. *Public Health Nutrition, 10*(4), 413–421. http://doi.org/10.1017/S1368980007248049

McDonagh, M. S., Selph, S., Ozpinar, A., & Foley, C. (2014). Systematic review of the benefits and risks of metformin in treating obesity in children aged 18 years and younger. *JAMA Pediatrics, 168*(2), 178–184. http://doi.org/10.1001/jamapediatrics.2013.42

McMurray, F., Church, C. D., Larder, R., Nicholson, G., Wells, S., Teboul, L., … Cox, R. D. (2013). Adult onset global loss of the FTO gene alters body composition and metabolism in the mouse. *PLoS Genetics, 9*(1), e1003166. http://doi.org/10.1371/journal.pgen.1003166

Merikangas, A. K., Mendola, P., Pastor, P. N., Reuben, C. A., & Cleary, S. D. (2012). The association between major depressive disorder and obesity in US adolescents: Results from the 2001–2004 National Health and Nutrition Examination Survey. *Journal of Behavioral Medicine, 35*(2), 149–154. http://doi.org/10.1007/s10865-011-9340-x

Messiah, S. E., Arheart, K. L., Lipshultz, S. E., & Miller, T. L. (2008). Body mass index, waist circumference, and cardiovascular risk factors in adolescents. *The Journal of Pediatrics, 153*(6), 845–850. http://doi.org/10.1016/j.jpeds.2008.06.013

Messiah, S. E., Arheart, K. L., Lipshultz, S. E., & Miller, T. L. (2011). Ethnic group differences in waist circumference percentiles among U.S. children and adolescents: Estimates from the 1999-2008 National Health and Nutrition Examination Surveys. *Metabolic Syndrome and Related Disorders, 9*(4), 297–303. http://doi.org/10.1089/met.2010.0127

Michalsky, M. P., Inge, T. H., Teich, S., Eneli, I., Miller, R., Brandt, M. L., … Buncher, R. C. (2014). Adolescent bariatric surgery program characteristics: The Teen Longitudinal

Assessment of Bariatric Surgery (Teen-LABS) study experience. *Seminars in Pediatric Surgery, 23*(1), 5–10. http://doi.org/10.1053/j.sempedsurg.2013.10.020

Mischel, W., Shoda, Y., & Rodriguez, M. L. (1989). Delay of gratification in children. *Science, 244*(4907), 933–938.

Morandi, A., Meyre, D., Lobbens, S., Kleinman, K., Kaakinen, M., Rifas-Shiman, S. L., … Froguel, P. (2012). Estimation of newborn risk for child or adolescent obesity: Lessons from longitudinal birth cohorts. *PloS One, 7*(11), e49919. http://doi.org/10.1371/journal.pone.0049919

National Health and Nutrition Examination Survey (NHANES). (2011). *Anthropometry procedures manual.* Retrieved from https://www.cdc.gov/nchs/data/nhanes/nhanes_11_12/Anthropometry_Procedures_Manual.pdf

Nederkoorn, C., Jansen, E., Mulkens, S., & Jansen, A. (2007). Impulsivity predicts treatment outcome in obese children. *Behaviour Research and Therapy, 45*, 1071–1075. http://doi.org/10.1016/j.brat.2006.05.009

O'Connor, E. A., Evans, C. V., Burda, B. U., Walsh, E. S., Eder, M., & Lozano, P. (2017). Screening for obesity and intervention for weight management in children and adolescents: Evidence report and systematic review for the US Preventive Services Task Force. *Journal of the American Medical Association, 317*(23), 2427–2444.

O'Neil, C. E., Byrd-Bredbenner, C., Hayes, D., Jana, L., Klinger, S. E., & Stephenson-Martin, S. (2014). The role of breakfast in health: Definition and criteria for a quality breakfast. *Journal of the Academy of Nutrition and Dietetics, 114*(12 Suppl), S8–S26. http://doi.org/10.1016/j.jand.2014.08.022

Ogden, C. L., Carroll, M. D., Kit, B. K., & Flegal, K. M. (2012). *Prevalence of obesity and trends in body mass index among US children and adolescents*, 1999-2010. *Journal of the American Medical Association, 307*(5), 483–490. http://doi.org/10.1001/jama.2012.40

Ogden, C. L., Carroll, M. D., Lawman, H. G., Fryar, C. D., Kruszon-Moran, D., Kit, B. K., & Flegal, K. M. (2016). Trends in obesity prevalence among children and adolescents in the United States, 1988–1994 through 2013–2014. *Journal of the American Medical Association, 315*(21), 2292–2299. http://doi.org/10.1001/jama.2016.6361

Park, M. H., Falconer, C., Viner, R. M., & Kinra, S. (2012). The impact of childhood obesity on morbidity and mortality in adulthood: A systematic review. *Obesity Reviews, 13*(11), 985–1000. http://doi.org/10.1111/j.1467-789X.2012.01015.x

Patton, J. H., Stanford, M. S., & Barratt, E. S. (1995). Factor structure of the Barratt impulsiveness scale. *Journal of Clinical Psychology, 51*(6), 768–774. http://doi.org/10.1002/1097-4679(199511)51:6<768::AID-JCLP2270510607>3.0.CO;2-1

Peirson, L., Fitzpatrick-Lewis, D., Morrison, K., Warren, R., Usman Ali, M., & Raina, P. (2015). Treatment of overweight and obesity in children and youth: A systematic review and meta-analysis. *CMAJ Open, 3*(1), E35–46. http://doi.org/10.9778/cmajo.20140047

Pereira, M. A., Erickson, E., McKee, P., Schrankler, K., Raatz, S. K., Lytle, L. A., & Pellegrini, A. D. (2011). Breakfast frequency and quality may affect glycemia and appetite in adults and children. *Journal of Nutrition, 141*(1), 163–168. http://doi.org/10.3945/jn.109.114405

Piernas, C., & Popkin, B. M. (2011). Increased portion sizes from energy-dense foods affect total energy intake at eating occasions in US children and adolescents: Patterns and trends by age group and sociodemographic characteristics, 1977-2006. *The American Journal of Clinical Nutrition, 94*(5), 1324–1332. http://doi.org/10.3945/ajcn.110.008466

Pollack, A. (2013, June 28). A.M.A. recognizes obesity as a disease. *The New York Times.* Retrieved from http://www.nytimes.com/2013/06/19/business/ama-recognizes-obesity-as-a-disease.html

Poti, J. M., & Popkin, B. M. (2011). *Trends in energy intake among US children by eating location and food source, 1977–2006. Journal of the American Dietetic Association, 111*(8), 1156–1164. http://doi.org/10.1016/j.jada.2011.05.007

Powell, L. M., & Nguyen, B. T. (2013). Fast-food and full-service restaurant consumption among children and adolescents: Effect on energy, beverage, and nutrient intake. *JAMA Pediatrics, 167*(1), 14–20. http://doi.org/10.1001/jamapediatrics.2013.417

Puder, J. J., & Munsch, S. (2010). Psychological correlates of childhood obesity. *International Journal of Obesity, 34*, S37–S43. http://doi.org/10.1038/ijo.2010.238

Quattrin, T., Roemmich, J. N., Paluch, R., Yu, J., Epstein, L. H., & Ecker, M. A. (2014). Treatment outcomes of overweight children and parents in the medical home. *Pediatrics, 134*, 290–297. http://doi.org/10.1542/peds.2013-4084

Ren, D., Zhou, Y., Morris, D., Li, M., Li, Z., & Rui, L. (2007). Neuronal SH2B1 is essential for controlling energy and glucose homeostasis. *The Journal of Clinical Investigation, 117*(2), 397–406. https://doi.org/10.1172/jci29417

Rogers, R., Eagle, T. F., Sheetz, A., Woodward, A., Leibowitz, R., Song, M., … Eagle, K. A. (2015). The relationship between childhood obesity, low socioeconomic status, and race/ethnicity: Lessons from Massachusetts. *Childhood Obesity, 11*(6), 691–695. http://doi.org/10.1089/chi.2015.0029

Sabin, M. A., Ford, A., Hunt, L., Jamal, R., Crowne, E. C., & Shield, J. P. (2007). Which factors are associated with a successful outcome in a weight management programme for obese children? *Journal of Evaluation in Clinical Practice, 13*(3), 364–368. http://doi.org/10.1111/j.1365-2753.2006.00706.x

Savoye, M., Nowicka, P., Shaw, M., Yu, S., Dziura, J., Chavent, G., … Caprio, S. (2011). Long-term results of an obesity program in an ethnically diverse pediatric population. *Pediatrics, 127*(3), 402–410. http://doi.org/10.1542/peds.2010-0697

Saxena, R., Hivert, M.-F., Langenberg, C., Tanaka, T., Pankow, J. S., Vollenweider, P., … Zhao, J. H. (2010). Genetic variation in GIPR influences the glucose and insulin responses to an oral glucose challenge. *Nature Genetics, 42*(2), 142–148. https://doi.org/10.1038/ng.521

Schlam, T. R., Wilson, N. L., Shoda, Y., Mischel, W., & Ayduk, O. (2013). Preschoolers' delay of gratification predicts their body mass 30 years later. *The Journal of Pediatrics, 162*(1), 90–93. http://doi.org/10.1016/j.jpeds.2012.06.049

Shrewsbury, V. A., Steinbeck, K. S., Torvaldsen, S., & Baur, L. A. (2011). The role of parents in pre-adolescent and adolescent overweight and obesity treatment: A systematic review of clinical recommendations. *Obesity Reviews, 12*(10), 759–769. http://doi.org/10.1111/j.1467-789X.2011.00882.x

Singh, A. S., Mulder, C., Twisk, J. W., van Mechelen, W., & Chinapaw, M. J. (2008). Tracking of childhood overweight into adulthood: A systematic review of the literature. *Obesity Reviews, 9*(5), 474–488. http://doi.org/10.1111/j.1467-789X.2008.00475.x

Smith, K. J., Gall, S. L., McNaughton, S. A., Blizzard, L., Dwyer, T., & Venn, A. J. (2010). Skipping breakfast: Longitudinal associations with cardiometabolic risk factors in the Childhood Determinants of Adult Health Study. *The American Journal of Clinical Nutrition, 92*(6), 1316–1325. http://doi.org/10.3945/ajcn.2010.30101

Smith, K. L., Straker, L. M., McManus, A., Fenner, A. A. (2014). Barriers and enablers for participation in healthy lifestyle programs by adolescents who are overweight: A qualitative study of the opinions of adolescents, their parents and community stakeholders. *BMC Pediatrics, 14*, 53. http://doi.org/10.1186/1471-2431-14-53

Spear, B. A., Barlow, S. E., Ervin, C., Ludwig, D. S., Saelens, B. E., Schetzina, K. E., & Taveras, E. M. (2007). Recommendations for treatment of child and adolescent overweight and obesity. *Pediatrics, 120*(Suppl 4), S254–S288. http://doi.org/10.1542/peds.2007-2329F

Speliotes, E. K., Willer, C. J., Berndt, S. I., Monda, K. L., Thorleifsson, G., Jackson, A. U., … Loos, R. J. (2010). Association analyses of 249,796 individuals reveal 18 new loci associated with body mass index. *Nature Genetics, 42*(11), 937–948. http://doi.org/10.1038/ng.686

Steinberg, L., Graham, S., O'Brien, L., Woolard, J., Cauffman, E., & Banich, M. (2009). Age differences in future orientation and delay discounting. *Child Development, 80*(1), 28–44. http://doi.org/10.1111/j.1467-8624.2008.01244.x

Swinburn, B. A., Sacks, G., Hall, K. D., McPherson, K., Finegood, D. T., Moodie, M. L., & Gortmaker, S. L. (2011). The global obesity pandemic: Shaped by global drivers and local environments. *The Lancet, 378*(9793), 804–814. http://doi.org/10.1016/s0140-6736(11)60813-1

Tanofsky-Kraff, M., Han, J. C., Anandalingam, K., Shomaker, L. B., Columbo, K. M., Wolkoff, L. E., … Yanovski, J. A. (2009). The FTO gene rs9939609 obesity-risk allele and loss of control over eating. *The American Journal of Clinical Nutrition, 90*(6), 1483–1488. http://doi.org/10.3945/ajcn.2009.28439

Tanofsky-Kraff, M., Yanovski, S. Z., Schvey, N. A., Olsen, C. H., Gustafson, J., & Yanovski, J. A. (2009). A prospective study of loss of control eating for body weight gain in children at high risk for adult obesity. *The International Journal of Eating Disorders, 42*(1), 26–30. http://doi.org/10.1002/eat.20580

Teixeira, P. J., Carraca, E. V., Marques, M. M., Rutter, H., Oppert, J. M., De Bourdeaudhjuij, I., … Brug, J. (2015). Successful behavior change in obesity interventions in adults: A systematic review of self-regulation mediators. *BMC Medicine, 13*, 84. http://doi.org/10.1186/s12916-015-0323-6

Temple, J. L., Legierski, C. M., Giacomelli, A. P., Salvy, S., & Epstein, L. H. (2008). Overweight children find food more reinforcing and consume more energy than do non-overweight children. *The American Journal of Clinical Nutrition, 87*, 1121–1127.

Theim, K. R., Sinton, M. M., Goldschmidt, A. B., Van Buren, D. J., Doyle, A. C., Saelens, B. E., … Wilfley, D. E. (2013). Adherence to behavioral targets and treatment attendance during a pediatric weight control trial. *Obesity, 21*(2), 394–397. http://doi.org/10.1002/oby.20281

The State of Obesity. (2017). *Overview.* Retrieved from https://stateofobesity.org/childhood-obesity-trends/

Thorndike, A. N., Riis, J., Sonnenberg, L. M., & Levy, D. E. (2014). Traffic-light labels and choice architecture: Promoting healthy food choices. *American Journal of Preventive Medicine, 46*(2), 143–149. http://doi.org/10.1016/j.amepre.2013.10.002

Thorndike, A. N., Sonnenberg, L. M., Riis, J., Barraclough, S. J., & Levy, D. E. (2012). A 2-phase labeling and choice architecture intervention to improve healthy food and beverage choices. *American Journal of Public Health, 102*(3), 527–533. http://doi.org/10.2105/AJPH.2011.300391

Treadwell, J. R., Sun, F., & Schoelles, K. (2008). Systematic review and meta-analysis of bariatric surgery for pediatric obesity. *Annals of Surgery, 248*(5), 763–776. http://doi.org/10.1097/SLA.0b013e31818702f4

Unger, T. J., Calderon, G. A., Bradley, L. C., Sena-Esteves, M., & Rios, M. (2007). Selective deletion of Bdnf in the ventromedial and dorsomedial hypothalamus of adult mice results in hyperphagic behavior and obesity. *The Journal of Neuroscience, 27*(52), 14265–14274. https://doi.org/10.1523/jneurosci.3308-07.2007

US Department of Health and Human Services & US Department of Agriculture. (2015). *2015–2020 Dietary guidelines for Americans.* 8th ed. Retrieved from http://health.gov/dietaryguidelines/2015/guidelines/

US Food and Drug Administration. (2003). *Xenical approval letter* (NDA 20-766/S-018). Retrieved from https://www.accessdata.fda.gov/drugsatfda_docs/appletter/2003/20766se5-018ltr.pdf

US Food and Drug Administration. (2010). *Drug safety communication: Completed safety review of Xenical/Alli (orlistat) and severe liver injury.* Retrieved from https://www.fda.gov/Drugs/DrugSafety/PostmarketDrugSafetyInformationforPatientsandProviders/ucm213038.htm

van den Berg, L., Pieterse, K., Malik, J. A., Luman, M., Willems van Dijk, K., Oosterlaan, J., & Delemarre-van de Waal, H. A. (2011). Association between impulsivity, reward responsiveness and body mass index in children. *International Journal of Obesity, 35*(10), 1301–1307. http://doi.org/10.1038/ijo.2011.116

Virudachalam, S., Long, J. A., Harhay, M. O., Polsky, D. E., & Feudtner, C. (2014). Prevalence and patterns of cooking dinner at home in the USA: National Health and Nutrition Examination Survey (NHANES) 2007-2008. *Public Health Nutrition, 17*(5), 1022–1030.9 http://doi.org/10.1017/S1368980013002589

Wardle, J., Guthrie, C. A., Sanderson, S., & Rapoport, L. (2001). Development of the Children's Eating Behaviour Questionnaire. *The Journal of Child Psychology and Psychiatry and Allied Disciplines, 42*(07), 963–970. http://doi.org/10.1111/1469-7610.00792

Wardle, J., Llewellyn, C., Sanderson, S., & Plomin, R. (2009). The FTO gene and measured food intake in children. *International Journal of Obesity, 33*(1), 42–45. http://doi.org/10.1038/ijo.2008.174

Waring, M. E., & Lapane, K. L. (2008). Overweight in children and adolescents in relation to attention-deficit/hyperactivity disorder: Results from a national sample. *Pediatrics, 122*(1), e1–e6. http://doi.org/10.1542/peds.2007-1955

Wennberg, M., Gustafsson, P. E., Wennberg, P., & Hammarstrom, A. (2015). Poor breakfast habits in adolescence predict the metabolic syndrome in adulthood. *Public Health Nutrition, 18*(1), 122–129. http://doi.org/10.1017/S1368980013003509

Whitaker, R. C., Wright, J. A., Pepe, M. S., Seidel, K. D., & Dietz, W. H. (1997). Predicting obesity in young adulthood from childhood and parental obesity. *New England Journal of Medicine, 337*(13), 869–873. http://doi.org/10.1056/NEJM199709253371301

White, B., Jamieson, L., Clifford, S., Shield, J. P., Christie, D., Smith, F., … Viner, R. M. (2015). Adolescent experiences of anti-obesity drugs. *Clinical Obesity, 5*(3), 116–126. http://doi.org/10.1111/cob.12101

Widenhorn-Muller, K., Hille, K., Klenk, J., & Weiland, U. (2008). Influence of having breakfast on cognitive performance and mood in 13- to 20-year-old high school students: Results of a crossover trial. *Pediatrics, 122*(2), 279–284. http://doi.org/10.1542/peds.2007-0944

Wildes, J. E., Marcus, M. D., Kalarchian, M. A., Levine, M. D., Houck, P. R., & Cheng, Y. (2010). Self-reported binge eating in severe pediatric obesity: Impact on weight change in a randomized controlled trial of family-based treatment. *International Journal of Obesity, 34*(7), 1143–1148. http://doi.org/10.1038/ijo.2010.35

Wilfley, D. E., Saelens, B. E., Stein, R. I., Best, J. R., Kolko, R. P., Schectman, K. B., … Epstein, L. H. (2017, October 30). Dose, content, and mediators of family-based treatment for childhood obesity: A multi-site randomized controlled trial. *JAMA Pediatrics.* Advance online publication. http://doi.org/10.1001/jamapediatrics.2017.2960

Wilfley, D. E., Staiano, A. E., Altman, M., Lindros, J., Lima, A., Hassink, S.G., … Cook, S. (2017). Improving access and systems of care for evidence-based childhood obesity treatment: Conference key findings and next steps. *Obesity, 25*(1), 16–29. http://doi.org/10.1002/oby.21712

Wilfley, D. E., Stein, R. I., Saelens, B. E., Mockus, D. S., Matt, G. E., Hayden-Wade, H. A., … Epstein, L. H. (2007). Efficacy of maintenance treatment approaches for childhood overweight: A randomized controlled trial. *Journal of the American Medical Association, 298*(14), 1661–1673. http://doi.org/10.1001/jama.298.14.1661

Wilfley, D. E., Vannucci, A., & White, E. K. (2010). Early intervention of eating- and weight-related problems. *Journal of Clinical Psychology in Medical Settings, 17,* 285–300. http://doi.org/10.1007/s10880-010-9209-0

Williams, N. A., Coday, M., Somes, G., Tylavsky, F. A., Richey, P. A., & Hare, M. (2010). Risk factors for poor attendance in a family-based pediatric obesity intervention program for young children. *Journal of Developmental and Behavioral Pediatrics, 31*(9), 705–712. http://doi.org/10.1097/DBP.0b013e3181f17b1c

Wolfe, B. M., Kvach, E., & Eckel, R. H. (2016). Treatment of obesity. *Circulation Research, 118,* 1844–1855. https://doi.org/10.1161/CIRCRESAHA.116.307591

World Health Organization. (2014). *Obesity and overweight* (Fact Sheet No. 311). Geneva, Switzerland: Author. Retrieved from http://www.who.int/topics/obesity/en/

Wrotniak, B. H., Epstein, L. H., Paluch, R. A., & Roemmich, J. N. (2004). Parent weight change as a predictor of child weight change in family-based behavioral obesity treatment. *Archives of Pediatric & Adolescent Medicine, 158*(4), 342–347. http://doi.org/10.1001/archpedi.158.4.342

Yang, J., Benyamin, B., McEvoy, B. P., Gordon, S., Henders, A. K., Nyholt, D. R., … Visscher, P. M. (2010). Common SNPs explain a large proportion of the heritability for human height. *Nature Genetics, 42*(7), 565–569. http://doi.org/10.1038/ng.608

Yildirim, M., van Stralen, M. M., Chinapaw, M. J., Brug, J., van Mechelen, W., Twisk, J. W., … Energy, C. (2011). For whom and under what circumstances do school-based energy balance behavior interventions work? Systematic review on moderators. *International Journal of Pediatric Obesity, 6*(2-2), e46–e57. http://doi.org/10.3109/17477166.2011.566440

Young, L. R., & Nestle, M. (2002). The contribution of expanding portion sizes to the US obesity epidemic. *American Journal of Public Health, 92*(2), 246–249. http://doi.org/10.2105/AJPH.92.2.246

Zeiss, A. M. (2016). Cognitive behavioral therapy as an integral component of interprofessional care. *Cognitive and Behavioral Practice, 23*, 441–445. http://doi.org/10.1016/j.cbpra.2016.01.004

Zeller, M. H., Reiter-Purtill, J., Ratcliff, M. B., Inge, T. H., & Noll, J. G. (2011). Two-year trends in psychosocial functioning after adolescent Roux-en-Y gastric bypass. *Surgery for Obesity and Related Diseases, 7*(6), 727–732. http://doi.org/10.1016/j.soard.2011.01.034

Zhang, X., Qi, Q., Zhang, C., Hu, F. B., Sacks, F. M., & Qi, L. (2012). FTO genotype and 2-year change in body composition and fat distribution in response to weight-loss diets: The POUNDS LOST trial. *Diabetes, 61*(11), 3005–3011. http://doi.org/10.2337/db11-1799

Zwintscher, N. P., Azarow, K. S., Horton, J. D., Newton, C. R., & Martin, M. J. (2013). The increasing incidence of adolescent bariatric surgery. *Journal of Pediatric Surgery, 48*(12), 2401–2407. http://doi.org/10.1016/j.jpedsurg.2013.08.015

8

Appendix: Tools and Resources

Session Outline

1. Weigh child and participating parent(s).

2. Record and graph weights.

3. Review self-monitoring and focus on what went well. (Offer praise)

4. Review weight change and link weight change to energy-balance behaviors.

5. Check for goals met. (Offer praise and problem solve challenges)

6. Create new plan for upcoming week.

D. E. Wilfley, J. R. Best, J. Cahill Holland, & D. J. Van Buren: *Childhood Obesity*　　　© 2019 Hogrefe Publishing

Summary of Weekly Goals

Day: _____   Date: ____/____/_____

Circle or Write In Your Weekly Goals

Weigh at Home	Eat 1,200-1,400 calories each day
Eat _____ or fewer RED foods per week	Plan for upcoming meals and physical activity
Eat 5+ GREEN servings of fruits and vegetables per day	Monitor all food and drink
Sleep ___ hours per night	Do physical activity for _____ minutes each day
Spend less than ___ hours per week doing RED activity	

Plan of Action – Weekly Intention

If:

Then:

D. E. Wilfley, J. R. Best, J. Cahill Holland, & D. J. Van Buren: *Childhood Obesity*   © 2019 Hogrefe Publishing

Planned Meals

Day: _____   Date: _____ / _____ / _____

Time/Hour Awake: _____   Time/Hour Fell Asleep: _____

Breakfast – Planned Time:	Amount	Calories	RED	GREEN
TOTAL BREAKFAST				
Lunch – Planned Time:	Amount	Calories	RED	GREEN
TOTAL LUNCH				
Dinner – Planned Time:	Amount	Calories	RED	GREEN
TOTAL DINNER				

Time	Snacks – Planned	Amount	Calories	RED	GREEN
	TOTAL SNACKS				
	TOTAL DAY				

Planned GREEN Physical Activity: _____ Min _____

D. E. Wilfley, J. R. Best, J. Cahill Holland, & D. J. Van Buren: *Childhood Obesity*   © 2019 Hogrefe Publishing

Eaten Meals

Day: _____   Date: ____ / ____ / _____

Time/Hour Awake: _____   Time/Hour Fell Asleep: _____

Breakfast – Eaten Time:	Amount	Calories	RED	GREEN
TOTAL BREAKFAST				

Lunch – Eaten Time:	Amount	Calories	RED	GREEN
TOTAL LUNCH				

Dinner – Eaten Time:	Amount	Calories	RED	GREEN
TOTAL DINNER				

Time	Snacks - Eaten	Amount	Calories	RED	GREEN
	TOTAL SNACKS				
	TOTAL DAY				

GREEN Physical Activity: _____   Min _____

Physical Activity Tracker

GREEN Activity

Day	Activity	Time	Intensity
		Total:	

RED Activity

Day	Activity	Time	Intensity
		Total:	

D. E. Wilfley, J. R. Best, J. Cahill Holland, & D. J. Van Buren: *Childhood Obesity*

Weekly Meal Planning and Physical Activity Worksheet

	Sunday	Monday	Tuesday	Wednesday	Thursday	Friday	Saturday
Breakfast approx. 300 – 500 Calories							
Lunch approx. 300 – 500 Calories							
Dinner approx. 300 – 500 Calories							
Snacks approx. 100 – 200 Calories							
Physical Activity							

D. E. Wilfley, J. R. Best, J. Cahill Holland, & D. J. Van Buren: *Childhood Obesity*

Pretreatment Assessment

Family ID _____   Interviewer _____   Date ___/___/_____

PARENT – Model of Support Strengths and Areas for Improvement Assessment

Therapist introduction to the assessment: "I would like to ask you some questions about your child's habits, your family and home environment, your child's friends, and the community in which you live, in each of the domains of the Model of Support. In our treatment program, we will focus on these levels (your child, your family, your child's peer network, and the surrounding community), as in each phase of treatment, there are things in those that can make it easier or harder to keep up with healthy eating and activity behaviors. We will identify strengths for your child and areas that could be improved in each level to help you and your child build permanent healthy eating and activity habits."

1. Self Environment

A. Eating Behaviors – Some people have certain traits that make them more vulnerable to having irregular eating patterns and overeating. These are called appetitive traits, and they can have a significance influence on weight. Does your child have any difficulty in the following areas?

		Never	Rarely	Sometimes	Often	Almost always
1.	Child engages in sneak eating behaviors	0	1	2	3	4
2.	Child has a hard time stopping eating once they start	0	1	2	3	4
3.	Child keeps eating even though they are full or have had enough	0	1	2	3	4
4.	Child feels badly about the amount of food they eat	0	1	2	3	4
5.	Child skips meals to avoid eating too much food	0	1	2	3	4
6.	Child continues to ask for and seek out opportunities to eat RED foods	0	1	2	3	4
7.	Child gets angry or frustrated when only healthy options are available or offered	0	1	2	3	4
8.	Child "grazes" on food throughout the day	0	1	2	3	4
9.	Child struggles with having smaller portions of foods	0	1	2	3	4

B. Internal State: Eating in Response to Emotions – Management of emotions can play a role in maintaining weight. Does your child eat in response to emotions?

	Never	Rarely	Sometimes	Often	Almost always
10. Child tends to eat when feeling afraid or scared	0	1	2	3	4
11. Child tends to eat when feeling sad or blue	0	1	2	3	4
12. Child tends to eat when feeling angry	0	1	2	3	4
13. Child tends to eat when feeling disappointed	0	1	2	3	4
14. Child tends to eat when feeling tired	0	1	2	3	4
15. Child tends to eat when feeling frustrated	0	1	2	3	4
16. Child tends to eat when feeling happy or excited	0	1	2	3	4
17. Child tends to eat when feeling bored	0	1	2	3	4
18. Child tends to eat when feeling lonely	0	1	2	3	4

Notes: _____

_____

_____

_____

STOP: Give Parent a Summary of Strengths and Areas for Improvement in Self Environment Domain. Discuss possible goals.

2. Family and Home Environment

A. Family Members – Each member of your immediate family plays a role in helping your child maintain healthy eating and activity habits.

19. Let's talk about the members of your family that live at home with your child and their relationship to your child. Also, it would be helpful to know if your child spends time in other households, either due to childcare arrangements (e.g., grandparents taking care of them) or due to custody arrangements (e.g., living with mom during week, and dad on the weekends). We can talk about how people in these other homes influence your child's eating and activity levels. For each person, how helpful are they with eating and activity goals (circle one): very helpful (++); a little helpful (+); make it a little difficult (–); or make it very difficult (– –)?

Name of immediate family member	Age	Relation to your child	Helps healthy eating or makes it difficult	Helps healthy physical activity or makes it difficult	Notes
			++ + − − −	++ + − − −	
			++ + − − −	++ + − − −	
			++ + − − −	++ + − − −	
			++ + − − −	++ + − − −	
			++ + − − −	++ + − − −	
			++ + − − −	++ + − − −	
			++ + − − −	++ + − − −	
			++ + − − −	++ + − − −	

B. Meal Regularity – How regularly does your child eat meals and snacks?

	Never	Rarely	Sometimes	Often	Almost always
20. Child eats three regular meals each day	0	1	2	3	4
21. Child eats breakfast	0	1	2	3	4
22. Child eats lunch	0	1	2	3	4
23. Child eats dinner	0	1	2	3	4
24. Is their meal pattern different on the weekend?	0	1	2	3	4
25. If meal pattern differs on the weekend, explain: _____					
26. Does your child eat snacks throughout the day?	0	1	2	3	4
27. Child eats a scheduled morning snack	0	1	2	3	4
28. Child eats a scheduled afternoon snack	0	1	2	3	4
29. Child eats a scheduled evening snack	0	1	2	3	4

D. E. Wilfley, J. R. Best, J. Cahill Holland, & D. J. Van Buren: *Childhood Obesity*   © 2019 Hogrefe Publishing

C. Sleep – Another area related to the regulation and the home environment is your child's sleep habits. Please describe your child's sleep habits.

		Never	Rarely	Sometimes	Often	Almost always
30.	Child gets between 9 and 11 hours of sleep each night	0	1	2	3	4
31.	Child wakes easily in the morning	0	1	2	3	4
32.	Child falls asleep without any difficulty	0	1	2	3	4
33.	Child follows a bedtime routine	0	1	2	3	4
34.	Child uses television as a way to fall asleep	0	1	2	3	4
35.	Child has a television in their bedroom	0	1	2	3	4
36.	Child uses texting/video/computer immediately before bed or to fall asleep	0	1	2	3	4
37.	Child has a well-established routine prior to going to bed	0	1	2	3	4

D. Family/Home Support: Healthy Eating – Now, I'm going to ask you about your child's environment and find out about their support at home for healthy eating. How often do the following behaviors occur?

		Never	Rarely	Sometimes	Often	Almost always
44.	Parent serves lean meats at family meals	0	1	2	3	4
45.	Parent serves vegetables with family meals	0	1	2	3	4
46.	Parent serves fruits and vegetables for snack at home	0	1	2	3	4
47.	Parent avoids serving RED food snack items at home	0	1	2	3	4
48.	Parent packs child lunch for school	0	1	2	3	4
49.	Family shops for groceries at least once a week	0	1	2	3	4
50.	How often are you eating meals at fast food or other restaurants?	0	1	2	3	4

D. E. Wilfley, J. R. Best, J. Cahill Holland, & D. J. Van Buren: *Childhood Obesity*   © 2019 Hogrefe Publishing

E. Family/Home Support: Physical Activity – Now, I'm going to ask you about your child's support for physical activity. How often does the following occur?

	Never	Rarely	Sometimes	Often	Almost always
51. Parents in home do physical activity with child	0	1	2	3	4
52. Siblings do physical activity with them (Check off: ☐ N/A – no siblings)	0	1	2	3	4
53. Child participates in teams or sports at school or in the neighborhood	0	1	2	3	4
54. Describe any physical activity equipment in or around the home that your child uses	0	1	2	3	4

Notes: _____

_____

_____

_____

STOP: Give Parent a Summary of Strengths and Areas for Improvement in Self Environment Domain. Discuss possible goals.

3. Peer Environment

A. Getting Along With Peers – I'm going to ask you some questions about your child's relationship with their peers.

	Never	Rarely	Sometimes	Often	Almost always
55. My child has trouble getting along with other kids	0	1	2	3	4
56. My child thinks that other kids do not want to be their friend	0	1	2	3	4
57. My child gets teased by other kids	0	1	2	3	4
58. My child has a difficult time keeping up physically with other kids	0	1	2	3	4

B. Peer Support for Healthy Eating and Activity

59.   List some of the friends in your child's peer network:

Name of friend	Age	Do they go to school together?	How often does your child see this friend?	Helps healthy eating or makes it difficult	Helps healthy physical activity or makes it difficult	Notes
		☐ Yes ☐ No	☐ Daily ☐ Weekly ☐ Monthly ☐ <Once/Month	++ + − −−	++ + − −−	
		☐ Yes ☐ No	☐ Daily ☐ Weekly ☐ Monthly ☐ <Once/Month	++ + − −−	++ + − −−	
		☐ Yes ☐ No	☐ Daily ☐ Weekly ☐ Monthly ☐ <Once/Month	++ + − −−	++ + − −−	
		☐ Yes ☐ No	☐ Daily ☐ Weekly ☐ Monthly ☐ <Once/Month	++ + − −−	++ + − −−	
		☐ Yes ☐ No	☐ Daily ☐ Weekly ☐ Monthly ☐ <Once/Month	++ + − −−	++ + − −−	
		☐ Yes ☐ No	☐ Daily ☐ Weekly ☐ Monthly ☐ <Once/Month	++ + − −−	++ + − −−	
		☐ Yes ☐ No	☐ Daily ☐ Weekly ☐ Monthly ☐ <Once/Month	++ + − −−	++ + − −−	
		☐ Yes ☐ No	☐ Daily ☐ Weekly ☐ Monthly ☐ <Once/Month	++ + − −−	++ + − −−	

Notes: _____

_____

_____

_____

STOP: Give Parent a Summary of Strengths and Areas for Improvement in Self Environment Domain. Discuss possible goals.

D. E. Wilfley, J. R. Best, J. Cahill Holland, & D. J. Van Buren: *Childhood Obesity*   © 2019 Hogrefe Publishing

4. Community Environment or Multiple Contexts

A. Extended Family – Now, we will talk about the community and other contexts surrounding your child, starting with your child's extended family.

Name of immediate family member	Age	Relation to your child	Helps healthy eating or makes it difficult	Helps healthy physical activity or makes it difficult	Notes
			++ + − − −	++ + − − −	
			++ + − − −	++ + − − −	
			++ + − − −	++ + − − −	
			++ + − − −	++ + − − −	
			++ + − − −	++ + − − −	
			++ + − − −	++ + − − −	
			++ + − − −	++ + − − −	
			++ + − − −	++ + − − −	

B. School – Now, tell me about your child's school.

	Never	Rarely	Sometimes	Often	Almost always
60. Child gets support from staff for healthy eating and physical activity behaviors	0	1	2	3	4
61. Child has the opportunity to choose healthy lunches at their school	0	1	2	3	4
62. Child has opportunity to get physical activity at school (gym, recess, etc.)	0	1	2	3	4

D. E. Wilfley, J. R. Best, J. Cahill Holland, & D. J. Van Buren: *Childhood Obesity*   © 2019 Hogrefe Publishing

C. Neighborhood – These questions are about your neighborhood. Does your child have access to the following?

63. Child has a grocery store within walking distance of home   ☐ Yes   ☐ No   If so, how many? _____

64. Child has a fast food restaurant in their neighborhood   ☐ Yes   ☐ No   If so, how many? _____

65. Child lives within walking distance of a park   ☐ Yes   ☐ No   If so, how many? _____

66. Child lives in a safe neighborhood (sidewalks/paths, safe to be outside)   ☐ Yes   ☐ No   If so, how many? _____

67. Child engages in physical activities in places within the neighborhood   ☐ Yes   ☐ No   If so, how many? _____

68. Child is active with friends and peers in the neighborhood   ☐ Yes   ☐ No   If so, which ones? _____
What activities do they do? _____

69. Parent has sought out community-based opportunities for child's and their own physical activities   ☐ Yes   ☐ No   If so, which ones? _____

Notes: _____

_____

_____

_____

STOP: Give Parent a Summary of Strengths and Areas for Improvement in Self Environment Domain. Discuss possible goals.

Model of Support Treatment Plan

SELF

Strengths   *Areas for Improvement*

_____   _____

_____   _____

_____   _____

FAMILY

Strengths   *Areas for Improvement*

_____   _____

_____   _____

_____   _____

FRIENDS

Strengths   *Areas for Improvement*

_____   _____

_____   _____

_____   _____

COMMUNITY/MULTIPLE CONTEXTS

Strengths   *Areas for Improvement*

_____   _____

_____   _____

_____   _____

Peer Commentaries

This brief volume is a gem! It is a comprehensive, up-to-date review of a major public health problem that provides a tremendous knowledge base about obesity in children for professionals new to the field and an extensive update for experienced clinicians and researchers. It covers the definition and measurement of obesity in children, with a thorough description of epidemiological, environmental, psychosocial, and genetic factors. Further, all aspects of treatment of childhood obesity – family-based lifestyle interventions, pharmacotherapy, and bariatric surgery – are thoroughly summarized.

Robert I. Berkowitz, MD, Professor of Psychiatry and Pediatrics, Center for Weight and Eating Disorders, Department of Psychiatry, University of Pennsylvania; Director of the Eating and Weight Disorders Research Program, Department of Child and Adolescent Psychiatry and Behavioral Sciences, Children's Hospital of Philadelphia, PA

With increasing rates of pediatric obesity and growing concern about its impact on the health of children, this book is an invaluable resource for professionals. This compact volume provides up-to-date information on the causes, consequences, assessment, and treatment of pediatric obesity, and an in-depth look at family-based treatment, an evidence-based approach to its management. This book should find a place on the bookshelf of all pediatric practitioners.

Marsha D. Marcus, PhD, Professor of Psychiatry and Psychology, University of Pittsburgh School of Medicine, PA

This book is must reading for health professionals who treat childhood obesity. In a concise and easy-to-read style, it provides an authoritative summary of scientific knowledge regarding the etiology, scope, and significance of childhood obesity. Moreover, it describes evidence-based procedures for diagnosis and treatment and provides a valuable compendium of tools to assist in clinical assessment and intervention. This remarkably useful book will be a great asset to clinicians, students, and anyone interested in the problem of childhood obesity.

Michael G. Perri, PhD, ABPP, is the Robert G. Frank Professor of Clinical and Health Psychology and Dean of the University of Florida College of Public Health and Health Professions, Gainesville, FL

This book is an excellent resource for pediatricians interested in preventing, managing, and treating childhood obesity. While easy to read, it is also thorough and complete in addressing everything clinicians need to know about childhood obesity. Topics covered range from the diverse causes of obesity, including rare genetic abnormalities, to a variety of proven methods for how to manage it, including family-based approaches, medications, and surgical interventions. This book will help all medical providers appreciate that childhood obesity is both a medical and social problem that needs critical attention and provides the tools and information that they need to deal with it.

Kimberly S. Heugele, DO, Diplomate of American Board of Pediatrics (ABP); Diplomate of American Board of Obesity Medicine (ABOM), St John's Well Child and Family Center, Lynwood, CA

Advances in Psychotherapy
Evidence-Based Practice

Developed and edited with the support of the
Society of Clinical Psychology (APA Division 12)

New
Titles

Editors

Danny Wedding, PhD, MPH, USA
Larry E. Beutler, PhD, USA
Kenneth E. Freedland, PhD, USA
Linda Carter Sobell, PhD, ABPP, USA
David. A. Wolfe, PhD, Canada

About the series

The *Advances in Psychotherapy* series provides therapists and students with practical, evidence-based guidance on the diagnosis and treatment of the most common disorders seen in clinical practice – and does so in a uniquely reader-friendly manner. Each book is both a compact "how-to" reference on a particular disorder, for use by professional clinicians in their daily work, and an ideal educational resource for students and for practice-oriented continuing education. The books all have a similar structure, and each title is a compact and easy-to-follow guide covering all aspects of practice that are relevant in real life. Tables, boxed clinical "pearls," and marginal notes assist orientation, while checklists for copying and summary boxes provide tools for use in daily practice.

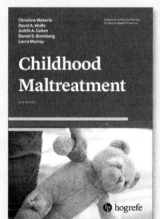

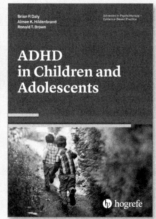

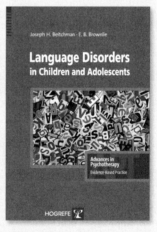

Volume 4
2nd ed. 2019, viii + 100 pp.
ISBN 978-0-88937-418-8

Volume 33
2016, viii + 90 pp.
ISBN 978-0-88937-412-6

Volume 28
2014, vi + 130 pp.
ISBN 978-0-88937-338-9

For a list of all current volumes, see next page.

www.hogrefe.com

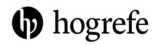 hogrefe

Advances in Psychotherapy

Prices: US $29.80 / € 24.95 per volume. Standing order price US $24.80 / € 19.95 per volume
(minimum 4 successive volumes) + postage & handling. Special rates for APA Division 12 and Division 42 members

www.hogrefe.com

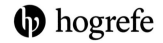

Earn 5 CE credits by reading volumes from the Advances in Psychotherapy book series

 New

How does it work?

Psychologists, therapists, and other healthcare providers can now earn 5 continuing education credits by simply reading volumes from the *Advances in Psychotherapy – Evidence-Based Practice* book series and taking an online multiple choice exam.

Readers can purchase each exam for $25 or access to the entire series of exams for $200. National Register members can take these exams free of charge.

This continuing education program is a partnership of Hogrefe Publishing and the National Register of Health Service Psychologists. The National Register of Health Service Psychologists is approved by the American Psychological Association to sponsor continuing education for psychologists and maintains responsibility for this program and its content.

Visit **www.hogrefe.com** to find out more!

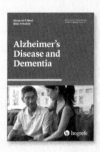 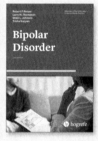 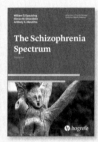 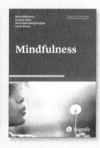 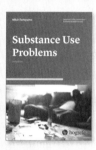

CE credits available for:
- ADHD in Adults
- ADHD in Children and Adolescents
- Alcohol Use Disorders
- Alzheimer's Disease and Dementia
- Binge Drinking and Alcohol Misuse Among College Students and Young Adults
- Bipolar Disorder, 2nd ed.
- Childhood Maltreatment
- Childhood Obesity
- Chronic Pain
- Depression
- Generalized Anxiety Disorder
- Headache
- Mindfulness

- Multiple Sclerosis
- Nicotine and Tobacco Dependence
- Obsessive-Compulsive Disorder in Adults
- Problem and Pathological Gambling
- Sexual Dysfunction in Men
- Sexual Dysfunction in Women
- Sexual Violence
- Social Anxiety Disorder
- Substance Use Problems, 2nd ed.
- Suicidal Behavior
- The Schizophrenia Spectrum, 2nd ed.
- Treating Victims of Mass Disaster and Terrorism
- Women and Drinking: Preventing Alcohol-Exposed Pregnancies

New titles are continually being added!

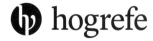 hogrefe

Quick and comprehensive information on psychotropic drugs for children and adolescents

Coming October 2018

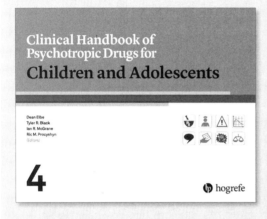

Dean Elbe / Tyler R. Black / Ian R. McGrane / Ric M. Procyshyn (Editors)

Clinical Handbook of Psychotropic Drugs for Children and Adolescents

4th edition 2019, iv + 395 pp.
+ 50 pp. of PDF patient / caregiver information sheets
US $99.80 / € 79.95
ISBN 978-0-88937-550-5
Also available as online version

This practical, spiral-bound book has become a standard reference and working tool for psychiatrists, pediatricians, psychologists, physicians, pharmacists, nurses, and other mental health professionals.

- Packed with unique, easy-to-read comparison charts and tables (dosages, side effects, pharmacokinetics, interactions...) for a quick overview of treatment options
- Succinct, bulleted information on all classes of medication: on- and off-label indications, side effects, interactions, pharmacodynamics, nursing implications, and much more – all you need to know for each class of drug
- Potential interactions and side effects summarized in comparison charts
- With instantly recognizable icons and in full color throughout, allowing you to find at a glance all the information you seek
- Clearly written patient and caregiver information sheets for download as printable PDF files

This book is a must for all mental health professionals working with children and adolescents who need an up-to-date, easy-to use, comprehensive summary of all the most relevant information about psychotropic drugs.

New in this edition:

- Drugs for ADHD thoroughly revised and updated
- Antipsychotics with many changes and additions, including fully revised lab tests/monitoring
- Antidepressants fully revised, including new sections on irreversible MAO-B inhibitor and serotonin modulator and stimulator (SMS)
- Hypnotics completely revised
- Mood stabilizers fully revised and a new toxicity comparison table added
- Drugs of abuse and treatment of substance use disorder comprehensively revised
- New unapproved treatments with significant updates, including: anti-inflammatories and NMDA agents in anxiety/OCD, cannabis use, and irritability of autism
- New agents include: TGAs N-arylpiperazine (brexpiprazole) and phenylpiperazine (cariprazine), hypnotics orexin receptor antagonist (hypnotic suvorexant) and selective melatonin agonist (tasimelteon), antidepressant bisarylsulfanyl amine (vortioxetine)
- New formulations and trade names

www.hogrefe.com

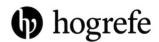